"This book fills the void in the traditional education of nutritionists. It offers an effective, compassionate and seasoned perspective, which will enhance, strengthen and define the crucial role of the nutritionist in the treatment of eating disorders. It is a user-friendly guide and will not only deepen every reader's perspective but will deepen the perspective of the entire nutritional counseling field. Bravo, Molly, and thank you for moving us forward."
Sondra Kronberg, MS, RD, CDN; author of <u>The Eating Disorder Learning/Teaching Handout Manual</u>; nutritional director, Eating Disorder Associates Treatment and Referral Centers, New York

"The next best thing to professional supervision with Molly. Educational, effective and empowering."
Suzanne Girard Eberle, MS, RD; author of <u>Endurance Sports Nutrition</u>

"Molly Kellogg's Counseling Tips for Nutrition Therapists is the pot of gold at the end of the dietitian rainbow! Filled with examples and practical solutions for the most demanding professional situations, Counseling Tips for Nutrition Therapists is THE book you will flip through before and after those nail-biting sessions. Even the most proficient nutrition authority will have something to learn from this comprehensive book."
Jessica Setnick, MS, RD; author, <u>The Eating Disorders Clinical Pocket Guide</u>, and founder, Eating Disorders Boot Camp: Training Workshop for Professionals

"An excellent, must-have tool for every dietitian counseling patients, whether a novice or a seasoned veteran. It is packed with practical case studies and tips, including helpful language to navigate tricky situations. Kellogg effectively bridges the tools of psycho-therapy and nutrition, honed by her years of experience as both a licensed therapist and dietitian."
Evelyn Tribole, MS, RD; co-author, <u>Intuitive Eating</u>

"… a wonderful resource written in clear, understandable language and presented in a format that encourages self-exploration. Readers can savor Molly's graceful and compassionate explanation of 25 common counseling situations. This Practice Workbook is a refreshing asset that has been enhanced by the honest and open case studies and contributions of many other dietitians that have worked with Molly over the years."
Megrette Hammond, co-founder of The Center for Mindful Eating and author of <u>Discover Mindful Eating: A Resource of Handouts for Health Professionals</u>

D1568845

"Finally, RDs have a guide to create meaningful sessions with our clients. The book is easy to read, to the point, and filled with relevant examples of how to manage day-to-day counseling situations, including how to handle personal questions, time boundaries, resistance, readiness to change (or lack thereof), staying on topic, clients who don't return ... all the situations I've wanted to know about so I could be a better counselor. Thank you, Molly."

Nancy Clark, MS, RD; author of <u>Nancy Clark's Sports Nutrition Guidebook</u>

Counseling Tips for Nutrition Therapists is a "must-read" for any dietitian who is interested in sharpening her/his counseling skills. Each chapter contains case studies and new approaches to address common situations. Useful tools that allow the dietitian to practice what is suggested are also included. A great resource for anyone conducting counseling."

Rebecca S. Reeves, DrPH, RD; assistant professor, managing director, Behavioral Medicine Research Center, Baylor College of Medicine; past president, American Dietetic Association

"Combining the best elements of case studies, practical applications, and self-practice (kind of like homework but more fun) – the book provides a theoretical framework that makes everything hang together. The quotes that serve as a springboard for each tip are ones you will want to incorporate into your own sessions with your clients because they serve to crystallize the concepts that follow. Kellogg combines both art and science in this book, and it is a wonderful blend."

Adrienne Ressler, MA, LMSW; national training director, The Renfrew Center Foundation; body image specialist

"A valuable resource for those of us working with clients who are struggling to heal diet trauma and/or recover from eating disorders. In easy-to-understand language, Kellogg provides the dietitian with ideas, tips and techniques needed to become more successful in difficult counseling situations. I recommend Counseling Tips to anyone who wants to improve their counseling skills, become more effective with clients, and more fully enjoy the counseling process."

Karin Kratina, PhD, RD, LD/N; co-author, <u>Moving Away From Diets</u>

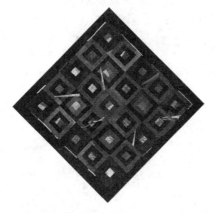

Counseling Tips for

Nutrition Therapists

Practice Workbook
Volume 1

Molly Kellogg, RD, LCSW

Kg Press
Philadelphia, PA

First Edition: Copyright 2006

Book Design: Sandy Gibson,
www.breezyhilldesigns.com
Copyeditor: Ellen Iwamoto
Cover Quilt Design: Melissa Sarris,
www.sarrisquilts.com

**Continuing Education Credits available
for Registered Dietitians.**
Details at www.mollykellogg.com

Kg Press
100 East Sedgwick St.
Philadelphia, PA 19119
215-843-8258
www.KgPress.com

ISBN 1933944021

CONTENTS

Introduction

Success is not a place at which one arrives,
but rather the spirit with which one
undertakes and continues the journey.
Alex Noble

A guideline can be thought of as a
signpost that leads us down the road—
until we reach the next sign.
Donald Altman

Nutrition counseling is challenging. Food behavior patterns are deeply entrenched. They are learned in families and reinforced over years into habits. Add to this, the tendency to turn to food for emotional reasons and the fact that food is essential for survival, and you have a recipe for behaviors that are very difficult to change. Our clients often know plenty about *what* to eat, but they need our help with *how* to do it. We are called on to be "change agents" in addition to the "educators" that we were trained to be.

Behavior change is hard. And we, whose profession it is to help others change, need support and guidance. This book is the product of my own frustration and the journey that resulted. With this book and others to follow I share with my nutrition colleagues the skills, language and approaches I have collected in a two-decade search for successful nutrition counseling.

The Author's Story

I entered the field of nutrition for several reasons. First, I loved science. Learning about biological processes was fascinating to me, and it seemed my interest would be unending. Nutrition science combined the hard sciences of biochemistry and physiology with the everyday practice of feeding ourselves. I wanted to make a difference in people's lives and knew that in nutrition I could do that.

After almost a decade working with pregnant women and families with young children, I started a private practice. I imagined helping clients to eat healthfully and to manage chronic conditions through diet. Very early in my practice, I became frustrated. I could tell my clients what to do, but most either did not change at all or adopted new behaviors only briefly before returning to old habits. Some clients described feeling helpless and compelled to eat even though they knew it was "wrong." When I worked with my first few clients with eating disorders, I finally could not deny that I, too, was helpless and needed more skills.

All my friends in counseling professions advised me to go to the Bryn Mawr School of Social Work. I became a licensed social worker in 1994 and worked as an outpatient psychotherapist for eight years while maintaining my part-time private practice in nutrition. Three years of gestalt therapy training deepened my professionalism and confidence.

My nutrition practice grew and became more rewarding as I integrated what I learned in the mental health field. I began to wonder whether any of my nutrition colleagues were as frustrated as I had been and whether I could pass on some of my knowledge to them. In early 2003, I felt inspired to write a brief article on self-disclosure for nutrition colleagues. It was a topic that, as a psychotherapist, I had always found compelling. I e-mailed it to a dozen or so local dietitians. They liked it, and I found myself interested in another topic and another and another. Soon the list of ideas for Tips was growing faster than I could write them. More and more nutrition professionals asked to be added to the mailing list, and in the spring of 2005, I transferred the list to an automated E-zine system. I still write one every month, and the list of ideas keeps growing. As of this writing, thousands of health professionals receive the Tips series.

In the last few years, I have added training workshops and professional supervision for nutrition professionals to my work. Readers of the series and workshop participants have asked for supporting materials. This workbook includes case studies from my practice and from the individual and group supervision I provide to health counselors around the country.

Please contact me.   I welcome feedback and suggestions for Tip topics.
molly@mollykellogg.com
www.mollykellogg.com

How to use this workbook

This book is designed to **wander around in**. You could read it cover-to-cover. But you will likely benefit more if you pick topics as they appeal to you. Read a chapter and then play with the ideas for a few days or weeks. Make notes in each chapter about what you have observed. Head back to a chapter that seems to call you again. When you circle back through a chapter, notice how much progress you have made! Professional growth and change flows best as an ongoing process of spiraling through observation, and experimentation over and over.

When you encounter **sample dialog** in a chapter you could use it as an exercise in creativity. Cover the page and peak at one line at a time. Each time you read what the client says, guess what you might say in response. Then read the suggested response and compare with yours.

A note about confidentiality

In case studies, client names and identifying information have been changed to protect privacy. When professionals have granted permission, their real names are used. Some have preferred to remain anonymous.

Acknowledgements

I would not have begun this project with out Lorraine Cohen, my life coach (www.powerfull-living.biz). She urged me to begin a newsletter and has provided emotional and practical support along the way.   She reinforces my growth process and makes it thoroughly enjoyable.

Lorraine referred me to Sandy Gibson, graphic designer (www.breezyhilldesigns.com), who is responsible for the gorgeous look of my website and this book.   I also found my virtual assistant, Susan

Schmidt (www.virtualassistanceonline.com), through Lorraine. Susan transcribed the recordings used in this book and handles administrative details too numerous to count. Ellen Iwamoto kept me in line with careful copyediting.

I appreciate all my colleagues who reviewed sections of the book: Susan D. Engle, MOE, RD; Maria Del Carmen Soler, MS, RD; Vicki Schwartz, RD; Laura Biron MBA, RD, CD; and Tracy Daly, MS, RD.

As I wrote these Tips month after month, many colleagues provided input on specific Tips catching unclear statements and adding useful insights. I hope I have remembered most of them here: Carolyn Bell, RD; Stephanie Brooks, MS, RD; Gretchen Newmark, RD; Marilyn Sarno, RD; Lauren Stern, MS, RD, CDN; and Monika Woolsey, MS, RD.

Jessica Setnick, MS, RD, has played a valuable role in my professional growth. We have grown and learned from each other as we develop training programs and home study programs together. She reviewed sections of this book and I always value her insightful, intelligent input.

Nutrition professionals all over the country allowed me to use their cases and our conversations about counseling process to add depth to these Tips. I am grateful to all whether their names are included or not.

I want to acknowledge Katherine Kurtz, LCSW, BCD, my clinical supervisor for 12 years. I model my supervision style on Katherine's and want her to know how much I value her contribution to my life and work. Cindy Shapiro, LCSW and Ellen Watson, LCSW, my partners in supervision for 10 years have taught me by example how to move forward in skills and depth of practice.

Last, but not least, my life partner, Jo Bennett, who edited early versions of the Tips, held me to high writing standards and provides daily support in my life.

Tip #1
Self-Disclosure

Reacting is an emotional reflex.
Response requires thought.
Gail Pursell Elliott

Self-disclosure is any sharing of information about yourself during a session. It ranges from mention of your family or where you vacation to your food preferences and eating habits, thoughts and feelings about your body, etc. This tip will address incidental self-disclosure that occurs during a session. Answering personal questions from a client is covered in Tip #18.

It can be very effective:

To **normalize** what the client is feeling, so she doesn't feel so alone or odd. "When I see a several-page restaurant menu, I find it overwhelming, too." Normalization can also be done by sharing (anonymously, of course) the experiences of other clients.

To **encourage** disclosure: "When I get to the end of my appetite and there is still delicious food on my plate, I often feel sad or disappointed. Do you ever feel something like that?"

To **broaden** the client's thinking: "For myself, I have found that a large, carbo-rich lunch tends to make me sleepy in the afternoon, so I choose not to feed myself that way on days I have lots to do." This can help a client see other ways to evaluate food rather than as only "good" or "bad."

To **model** more caring ways to treat oneself: When you make an error such as double scheduling or need to correct some information you gave the client, show that you can apologize, forgive yourself and move on. I often use phrases such as: "God isn't finished with me yet," or "Boy, I am a work-in-progress, aren't I?" We can choose to model self-forgiveness, especially with clients who struggle with perfectionism.

Cautions about use of self-disclosure:

It is best used *extremely* sparingly; once you've said it, you can't take it back. You may not be aware of how powerful self-disclosure can be to our clients. If you've been in therapy, remember when your therapist self-disclosed (if she did at all). Or remember how vividly you remember something you knew about a beloved teacher's personal life. When you share your personal experience or anything about your life, assume it will come across more strongly than you imagine.

Always use it **in service of the client**: Before self-disclosing, pause to ask yourself whether this information will help the client in an immediate way or whether it feels important to *you* to say it. For some of us, it's just the way we tend to converse. Counseling is different from everyday conversation. Self-disclosure is a powerful tool to be used deliberately. Decreasing self-disclosure in sessions can direct the tone away from chatting and toward a professional, effective relationship. Self-disclosure tends to shift the focus onto you. Here's a simple test: If you can maintain focus on the client while sharing your story, it's probably appropriate. If you become focused on the story, it's not.

Sometimes we talk about ourselves **to express care and understanding to a client**. This may be appropriate when conversing with a friend, but in a session, it's best to show you care in other ways.

Self-disclosure may work well with **one client but not another**. To best use your self-disclosure, the client needs to run your advice or modeling through her "gut" and either accept or reject it, depending on what is best for her. A low-functioning client who has a poorly formed sense of self is incapable of doing this. With a client who is an extreme caretaker, there is the danger you will encourage her to shift into being a caretaker for you. So, avoiding self-disclosure with less healthy clients is a wise choice.

Effective use of self-disclosure includes taking into account the stage of work with a client. Generally it's better to err on the side of caution at first with any client until you know her better. Sharing a bit of your experience may be a powerful tool **when the client is ready for it,** but harmful if done too soon.

If you are not sure how your self-disclosure was received, ask. "**What was it like** that I shared that with you?" If the client tells you of an association she had to your story, it likely moved the treatment along. If not, this is a clue to contain self-disclosure with her in the future.

Look for guidance:

It takes **experience to learn** when it's appropriate to self-disclose. If you're unsure in the moment, don't disclose and then jot it down to bring up in supervision or with a colleague you trust. If you find yourself self-disclosing more than once or twice a session, look at what it seems to do for you. Experiment with letting it go and see what happens.

Case Study: Self-Disclosure

This case is from my practice. Over the years, I have noticed that with certain clients I feel a strong urge to share about myself, but, with others, I feel less inclined to. Earlier in my practice, I would just respond to my inclination and share about myself if I believed it would be helpful to the client and if I felt like it.

A number of years ago, I noticed a stronger than usual urge to share about myself with a particular client. She was about my age, came from a similar background and was enjoyable to be with. I would even think of her after sessions and imagine sharing with her what was going on in my life. I knew this was a sign that I needed to work on this in supervision, so I brought the case to the supervision group I attend twice a month. The supervisor asked me what was different about this client for me at this particular time. After some exploration, I realized that my urge to talk about myself reflected my desire to be her friend. I liked her a lot, and from what I learned about her, we had a lot in common. I also realized that I was feeling lonely at that point in my life and needed more friends. I knew that she did not need me as a friend. She needed me as a nutritionist as she struggled with her relationship with food. If I tried to make the relationship more like a friendship, I would be of less value to her. I felt disappointed that I would not be able to enjoy a friendship with her and also knew what was best for her. I was then able to go back into our sessions with a renewed perspective on my role. I got over my disappointment in a week or so. I also took the clue about my needs and went out looking for more friends outside my work!

I now make use of these clues in client sessions. If I find myself wanting to share more than just a little about myself with a client, I work to sort it out. It could simply mean that I have a lot in common with this client and he or she would have made a good friend if we had met in a different context. Sometimes it is an indication that the client wants me to be a friend. If I suspect this is true, I set appropriate boundaries to keep the relationship professional. In the early years of my practice, I was tempted to self-disclose when I felt insecure about being able to connect with a client. I now keep my "self-disclosure filter" on tight enough that I don't do this, but I still feel the tug at times. I can choose to use this "tug" to inform me that I may not be connecting well with this person yet and find professional, effective ways to connect.

Practice Steps: Self-Disclosure

1. What is your natural style of self-disclosure? Spend a week or so just noticing what happens. In client sessions, how often do you tend to mention something about yourself or your food habits? What types of things do you share? What effect do these moments have on you? Do they help you stay focused on your client or distract you? Carefully observe your clients' reaction to your disclosures. Do they seem to incorporate them in useful ways?
2. It may be useful for you to observe other professionals. When you go to your doctor, accountant or therapist, look for examples of self-disclosure. If you find some, what is your reaction? Do they aid the process or distract?
3. If you tend to use self-disclosure more than once or twice in a session, try an experiment. Choose a block of clients. For example, one whole day or week, or several specific clients. In those sessions, contain all impulses to self-disclose and find other ways to accomplish each of your intentions. Expect it to feel awkward at first. What happens? Does it feel as if you are being any more or less effective? Does rapport seem stronger, weaker or just different?

4. You can use your eyes to assist you in staying focused on your client while self- disclosing. When you offer a brief piece from your life in the service of your client, it is easy to maintain eye contact with your client. If you notice that you break eye contact while telling your story, this likely means that you have gone too far.

My Experiments With Self-Disclosure:

What I observe:

_____
_____
_____
_____
_____
_____
_____
_____
_____

How I will experiment:

_____
_____
_____
_____
_____
_____
_____
_____
_____
_____

Tip #2
Using Your Client's Name

Everything has something to teach you.
Wayne Dyer

Some counseling concepts are big and important. This one is a simple idea, but it can be powerful.

Saying your client's name selectively tends to have the same effect that underlining or using italics does in text. It gets her attention and highlights what you are about to say. Think of the times people use your name and the effect it has on you.

Some examples:

You realize that she just said something important that reflects a **theme in your work** and you think she's missing its importance: "Hold on a minute, Sarah, let me see if I understand what you are saying. Every time you eat a food you call "bad," you feel guilty and then binge for the next few hours. Is that how it goes?"

You want to **reinforce some new behavior** that seems to be going in a healthy direction: "John, that's great! You've tested your blood sugar consistently for a week. Let's see how we can use that to help you feel better."

You realize you need to **shift gears** in the session because you and your client are off track: "You know, Joan, We could probably talk about that all day. I'm finding myself wondering if we are getting to what you really need today."

A caution:

It will lose its power if you use it **too often**. I generally don't say a client's name more than once or twice a session.

For a client who carries a lot of shame, it is possible that saying her name will trigger feelings of being judged or criticized. Watch for the response when you say her name. If it simply gets her attention and focus, you're probably on target. If the client gets quiet and you seem to lose her for a few minutes, you may need to back off and use her name in only the most empathetic contexts.

Practice Steps: Using Your Client's Name

1. First, just notice how you tend to use (or not) your client's name. How often do you find yourself saying it and in what contexts? Tally up all the examples for a sample of clients. Note the clients' reaction.
2. Take a look at the examples and ask yourself if the frequency seems about right. If so, you could play around with when you use it, doing it more deliberately.
3. If you find that you never say a client's name, experiment with using it once or twice each session for a period of time and notice the results.

My Experiments With Using My Client's Name:

What I observe:

_____
_____
_____
_____

How I will experiment:

_____
_____
_____
_____

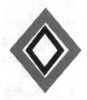

Tip #3
Behavioral Experiments

Do not be too timid and squeamish about your actions. All life is an experiment. The more experiments you make the better. What if they are a little coarse, and you may get your coat soiled or torn? What if you do fail, and get fairly rolled in the dirt once or twice. Up again, you shall never be so afraid of a tumble.

Ralph Waldo Emerson

I am always doing that which I can not do, in order that I may learn how to do it.

Pablo Picasso

"Experiments" in a counseling setting are behavior trials that are designed to gain further information for you and your client. They are used extensively by gestalt-trained therapists and fit beautifully with nutrition counseling.

Examples of experiments in nutrition counseling:

With a client working to recover from dieting, you notice that she is holding onto the "no food between meals" rule and is so hungry by her lunch break that she eats beyond satisfaction. You suggest an experiment to find out what would happen if she had a small morning snack. You help her think of some snack ideas and ask her to alternate days with a snack and days without, so she can clearly see differences.

With a **bulimic** client who says she is ready to decrease her reliance on purging, you suggest an experiment to be done just once that will put a step between the urge and the behavior. Maybe it would be writing in her journal or leaving a quick message on your voice mail. With this kind of experiment, it would be important to explain that stopping the behavior is not the goal, it's only to find out what happens when a little pause is inserted before it. Also, urge her to do it only once before you next see her.

You have a weight-loss client who wishes to address his "**clean plate syndrome**." Help him design an experiment to find out more about what this is all about for him. Maybe it would be to leave one tiny bite at each meal for a day and listen to the self-talk about it. Maybe it would be putting less on the plate one night, and timing a 15-minute wait for a second serving. Of course, this classic experiment works only if it is clear that the seconds are indeed allowed and that the goal is not to avoid them.

Some advantages:

Experiments encourage your client to be a careful observer of **process and outcome**, always important steps in real change. With much of nutrition counseling, the answers are mostly inside the client. So approaching your work as a series of experiments helps keep your mind-set in that curious state that allows the work to progress organically.

They are powerful because they are **approached as data collection** rather than as a new behavior you are telling the client to do. Many people can do something once if they don't think they will then have to do it for the rest of their lives. One result may be that they like the outcome and decide to continue. If you present the idea with a curious mind-set (even if you have a pretty good idea of what will happen) and urge the client to approach it with an open mind, the data collected will be most useful. And you may be surprised!

This approach is particularly useful with **risk-averse people**. Anxious clients (and that's most folks with eating disorders) may be more likely to try a new behavior that is presented as an experiment. Make sure to keep the focus on data collection.

Some cautions:

Tell your client that experiments often provide surprising data. **Whatever happens** will be useful, even if she finds herself not running the experiment. That would be really interesting! Explore that outcome as curiously as you do the data from the experiments that run as planned. Just as with scientific experiments, some are run to confirm previous work and some are exploratory.

Some clients need **help with the data collection process.** This can be particularly true with eating-disorder clients. Often their current system of data collection is very narrow (for example, looking only at weight changes). Many will still need that obsessive data for a while. Encourage expanding their observations to include: how their energy was after that food, how it tasted, what others said (or didn't say), how long it took for the anxiety to drift away, etc.

Experiments can be playful. Have fun!

Case Study: A Dietitian Learns New Skills by Experimenting

Suzanne Boos, RD, of Littleton, Colorado, attended one of my training workshops, and at the one-month follow-up conference call, I asked what she had taken from it. She first described a dilemma she had long struggled with. She had often wondered if she was confrontational enough with some clients, especially in the area of weight loss. When clients returned and had not done what was agreed on, she would assume that they already knew what they should have done and had beat themselves up enough. So she would take a more forgiving approach, pointing out that self-criticism doesn't lead to change and suggesting that they be good to themselves and try again. After sessions, she would wonder if this was what they wanted and was most useful for them. Maybe some clients just wanted accountability.

After the Counseling Intensive workshop, she wanted to incorporate Motivational Interviewing techniques, so she put some of the questions on her desk where she could easily see them.

She began to glace at them to help her launch into exploring what is important to clients and how confident they are. She found it quite awkward at first and was fearful that clients would feel threatened. To her surprise, her clients seemed to like it and they became more thoughtful about their behavior. She noticed that the very questions that had seemed so scary to her simply caused her clients to step back and take a look at their motivations and what was getting in the way of changing.

When she began the experiment of throwing in Motivational Interviewing questions, she had no idea she would be addressing her dilemma about confrontation. She discovered that the dilemma had melted away while she focused on her experiment. This is a magnificent example of surprising outcomes when we have the courage to try something new.

Case Study: An Accidental Experiment

Sometimes a client runs an experiment unintentionally, and it is useful to reframe it for him. This happened for a client, Jim, who was working on losing weight. He struggled with his portions at dinner. He knew he was eating more than he needed because he felt overly full after most dinners. He had tried putting less on his plate but said he felt deprived because it looked so meager. He would eat it fast and then quickly get seconds. He was not able to tolerate waiting 15 minutes for seconds as I suggested. One day, he came into my office pleased with himself. He told me that a few nights before he had filled his plate with the "right" portion but knew he would get seconds. Just as he finished the first helping, the phone rang. It was a favorite cousin he had not talked to in quite a while. Twenty minutes later, when he got off the phone, he headed to get more food but realized he did not feel at all hungry and so put away the leftovers. Jim was so surprised and pleased that he decided the next night he would make a phone call after his first helping to see if the same thing happened. He told me that it didn't work because the person he called was not home.

I congratulated Jim on deciding to expand on his accidental experiment to learn more about his process at dinner. Rather than seeing the second night as a failure, I suggested we look at it as a very interesting experiment. Jim had liked science in high school, so, using the language of experiments, we "collected data" first. He could see that the first night was so successful because he had been distracted for 20 minutes by a pleasant experience. The second night, it was only a minute or so, and he ended up disappointed. Using the results from those two evenings, we designed some more experiments. I urged him to try several combinations and to wait to make final conclusions. He decided to develop a list of people to call and plan to keep calling until he had talked for at least 15 minutes. Fortunately, he has a large family and many friends. He worried that some nights he might not feel like talking, so he came up with a list of other things he might do in that 15 minutes. Some of them sounded to me like chores. I know that many people use food to avoid unpleasant tasks, but I decided not to steer him away from those. I only pointed out that his list of choices had wonderful variety and suggested he carefully observe, as a scientist does, if there is any difference in the effectiveness of the various options.

When he reported on his experiments I was surprised to hear that the distracting activities that had sounded like chores to me were the most effective ones for him. The sense of achievement he got from accomplishing a small task gave him a lift that contributed to his feeling of success. I was glad that I had let him design the experiment and had kept my suggestions to a minimum. By the time he had run all of the experiments, he had experienced smaller dinners often enough to have broken his long-standing habit. He liked my suggestion of maintaining a "scientist's mind" about his dinnertime for at least another month to see what else he could learn.

Sample Dialog: Experiments

Notice that I work with the client to design the experiment rather than handing it to him.

Jack: I really should take my lunch to work. The stuff I can buy around my job is all greasy.

Molly: Have you ever done it before?

Jack: No, it's just so easy to go out and get something.

Molly: So you don't even know if you would like it or not?

Jack: Well, I guess it might be OK. I would save money. That would be great.

Molly: Hmmm. This sounds like a perfect situation for an experiment. Would you be willing to try it out a few times to gather more information about it?

Jack: Sure. I could do it next week.

Molly: Well, what would you want to learn from the experiment? Maybe to see if you do actually save money? How much trouble it is? If the food tastes OK? What else?

Jack: I do wonder whether my co-workers will give me a hard time.

Molly: Oh, do they tend to do that, and would that make it not worth it?

Jack: They do tease about some things. I could probably come up with something to say back.

Molly: Do you want to do one trial run first rather than committing to every day?

Jack: Good idea. I know I will have leftovers on Monday since my wife always cooks a lot on Sundays. I could just tell people my wife made me bring it. That might work.

Molly: Sounds like you have an initial experiment to try. Stay curious about how it goes and we can talk about it next time.

Next Session:

Molly: How did your experiment go?

Jack: Well, I certainly learned a lot! For one thing, bringing leftovers didn't work because we don't have a microwave and I don't like them cold. It turned out that the guys didn't get on my case. One even said he admired me for wanting to save money.

Molly: Oh, so this was a useful experiment. Anything else?

Jack: Well, my wife offered to make a sandwich one day and that was OK, except it didn't seem like enough.

Molly: Enough?

Jack: Well, I guess it was enough because I wasn't hungry until I got home, but it just seemed too simple. When I eat out, they give you chips and pickles.

Molly: What could you (or your wife) add to the bag to make it seem more full?

Jack: It wouldn't need to be much, just something. What do you think?

Molly: How would some baby carrots or pickles or a piece of fruit sound to you?

Jack: I like all of those.

Molly: Imagine for a moment being at work and opening the bag and seeing a sandwich and carrots and a piece of fruit. How does that feel?

Jack: That seems fine. I just need more than one thing.

Molly: So we've discovered some really useful stuff doing this experiment!

Jack: Yeah. I'll ask my wife to make that kind of lunch most days next week and I'll let you know how it goes. Now can we talk about eating out?

Molly: Sure. Another great opportunity to set up an experiment!

Language That Encourages Experimentation:

"I'll be darned, that's interesting! I wonder what we can learn from that."

"I wonder what would happen if you were to... Are you curious, too?"

"Well, whatever happens this week, it will be useful for us in figuring out how to help you make these changes."

"I wonder what your day (or life) would be like if you were to..."

"What would be useful to notice when you try this out? Do you want to take notes about things like how long it takes, if you do have more energy that day, or what people say to you about it? What else might you want to gather information about to make this experiment most useful?"

"I hear that you don't feel ready to try this even once. I wonder what we can learn from just imagining doing it. If you were to find something to distract you after eating a lot so you wouldn't purge, what would it be? What would be strong enough? Let's say you got interrupted right after a binge and were not able to purge for a few hours. What do you imagine would happen? How long do you imagine it would be before the urge lessened?"

Some clients don't like the idea of experiments because it sounds too scientific. If you get this feedback, try other metaphors such as a "dress rehearsal" or "trial run" or "pilot project" or "information-gathering expedition."

Practice Steps: Experiments

1. If you use the experimental process now, notice what roles you and your client take. Are you the "scientist" and the client the "guinea pig"? If so, try out some of the language in the box to shift your role to "consultant scientist" and your client's role to that of "lead researcher."

2. If you don't employ this technique yet, search for opportunities to suggest that your clients experiment. After trying it out at least five times and observing what happens over time in each case, evaluate the results.

My Experiments with Behavioral Experiments:

What I observe:

_____
_____
_____
_____
_____
_____

How I will experiment:

_____
_____
_____
_____
_____
_____
_____

Tip #4
Asking Your Client for Ideas and Direction

You cannot teach a man anything; you can only help him find it within himself.
Galileo

I know we are the **nutrition experts**. We've been saying that for decades. But we are not the experts about some things, our clients are, and we need to ask them.

Some examples:

- ♦ "What do you most want to achieve through nutrition counseling? **What matters** to you?"

- ♦ To find the preconceived notions of what you can do for the client: "What do you hope **I will do for you**? What role do you need me to take here?"

- ♦ "I hear that you want to be more physically active. **What ideas** do you have?" This one saves time because you find out what has not worked for your client and what may feel feasible.

- ♦ "Are you asking me for suggestions about this?" or "I have some ideas about that. Are you interested?" Consider asking this when you are about to launch into your **advice-giving mode**. If you get a "yes," you will have your client's attention. You may get a "yes" that comes with qualifications so you can tailor your advice. Or you might get a "no" and avoid wasting everyone's time. How do you feel when someone gives you advice you didn't ask for?

- "We have talked about lots of possible changes. What do you want to **address first?**" This is helpful when there seem to be lots of directions your work could go. Your opinion about how best to proceed is only one of two in the room. Consider bringing your client in on the choice and see what happens.

- When you sense you've just **lost your client** or when you've been talking for a while: "Let's see, where were we?" "Is this what you need?" "Are you getting what you came for?"

- "I can tell you are feeling frustrated (or stuck or sad). **How can I support you** right now?" This is a good one when you're feeling clueless or powerless to help. She may indeed tell you exactly what you can do. Or she may tell you that simply listening is enough.

Advantages:

Asking your client for direction several times during a session reminds you to focus on the **client's perspective**/needs/abilities. It sends the message (and reminds you) that many of the answers are in the client.

With passive or resistant clients, it encourages them to **take an active role**. When you feel you are working harder than your client, it's time to check in.

It slows down a session and invites **a shift of gears**. Frankly, I often find that the response is not precisely an answer to what I asked, but a discovery in the client that came out of the opening my question provided.

If you wonder after a session whether you did the best you could, this periodic check-in helps **reassure** you about being on track.

Finally, it helps you **stay connected**. A relationship supports the process of change. Checking in with your client nurtures the relationship. A client who feels connected with you is more apt to come for a return appointment.

Cautions:

I can't think of any.

Case Study: Asking Clients for Direction

This topic came up one day on a supervision conference call:

Kathee Varner, RD: A lot of what I do comes from the intuitive side. What does this person need? What is this person asking for? So I think in reviewing the sessions in my mind, a question keeps coming up: "What was my intention there?" Was that meeting her intention or what she needed? Was that the best direction?

Molly: Do you actually talk about these questions out loud with the client? Do you ever shift gears and say, "Jane, now hang on a minute. Is what we're doing right now what you need?" or "I realize we have 10 minutes left. Are we getting to what you needed?"

Kathee: Rarely. That's a good idea.

Molly: It takes shifting gears, doesn't it? It's not easy doing that, especially if you're used to working intuitively and feel comfortable with it. It's like being in a stream that's flowing gently and you're just floating along and it's lovely. And in order to get up onto the shore to look at the bigger picture, it's a big effort. You have to paddle over to the side and grab a tree. It can feel jarring. Does that feel like it would be hard for you to do?

Kathee: No, I just think I need to remember to do it more often. I find clients don't offer the information. In fact, a client may deliberately withhold information unless you are good at asking questions. I have routine questions I ask that help me to uncover things. But if the question is not asked, the information doesn't get offered. I understand their fear and need to withhold information.

Molly: You can't read the client's mind, and they can't read yours. It is more likely that the useful tough information will come out if there is a periodic shifting of gears and stepping back or climbing up the tree or whatever image you want to use. An experiment is occurring to me, Kathee, if you're interested. You could play around with, in every single session for a week, throwing in some process comments or questions. Some stepping back and asking the client to paint a bigger picture. Every single session once or twice. How would that be?

Kathee: That would be a great idea. Could we go through some questions that might be asked?

Molly: There's the classic, "How are we doing now, Jane? Are we getting at what you need today?" There are also times where you could own up to needing to refocus. For example, "Can we hold on for a minute? I'm having this feeling that I might be missing something. I need to back up and look at the big picture. Can you help me? Now, what was it we were wanting to focus on in a broader sense? We've gotten off on this wonderful, interesting tangent, but I want to make sure it's where we need to go." Here I'm owning up to my part of needing to take a step back.

Gale Welter, MS, RD, CSCS: I had something like this happen recently. I've been unpacking more and being quiet. I'll ask a question and then be quiet. I also ask more often, "Is there something else?" That generally works well. I was talking to this client, and it drifted like you were saying, and I saw it. I knew what we were doing. For some reason, I said, "OK, we're about 20-30 minutes into our time, I think I know what we're doing here, but could you just tell me again what you wanted to accomplish today?" And I heard an entirely different thing than I thought and I said, "Oh my gosh, I am so glad I asked you." I had the wrong idea, and it was really empowering for both of us that I stopped and asked.

Molly: Let me point out to you, Gale, what you did. You made "I – You" contact with her. You said *I* would like *you* to tell *me*. When you ask that kind of question, you're asking for authentic, real interaction by bringing yourself in. You really wanted to know. You needed it. That's an example of a stance to take when you do this stepping back and checking in. Kathee, do you feel like you need more?

Kathee: I think I'll just take that piece for right now.

Robin Millet, MS, RD, CDN: I'm thinking of a client of mine to try this approach with. I struggle because she gives me so little. I probe, and she gives nothing. I'm not sure how to play this out with someone like that.

Molly: With a client who is depressed, or very young, or a people-pleaser, there's not a lot of *you* there for the "I – You" interaction. The client isn't very present. That's why you're feeling that it's not going to yield much if you ask her self to speak to your self, because there isn't much self there. Robin, your intuition is telling you something useful.

Robin: Even her therapist is having the same problem with her. I've done what I can with her.

Molly: So you and the therapist both notice that this patient has lots of walls protecting something. We have to assume that there's a pretty awful history for her to put up walls like that. You feel like you're boxed in and you can't get anywhere. I see that reticence as an expression of health. If someone has a lot of shame left over from trauma, she's going to need to go really slowly and step-by-step. To do it all at once she would be flooded, and she knows that at least unconsciously. She doesn't want to be totally flooded with feelings and be a puddle on the floor. Allowing her to go really slow and titrate how fast the work goes is often the only way to do it. It can mean that your sessions with her are really short. Maybe even 15 minutes or that the only actual talking about nutrition is 5 or 10 minutes. The rest would be talking about movies or something light that would bracket the work. Having a safe space around the scary stuff is what eventually can allow the scary stuff to come out. This is a model of working with trauma. It's excruciatingly slow. Your role as a dietitian can be having the patience to just do teeny little pieces. These clients are often not able to be clear with you about what they need. You may find it works better to take direction from the therapist.

Robin: So, should I give up asking her for direction?

Molly: I wouldn't completely give up. You may just need to do it with very minor choices such as which chairs you each sit in or which food journal form works best for her.

Case Study: Asking a Client About Backing Off

Marcia Dadds, MS, RD, of New York, shares this wonderful example of the power of checking in with a client about process in the session:

> I wanted to tell you what happened after I attended the Counseling Intensive last week. As a result of all the looking at resistance, I realized I had pushed an anorexic client harder than I usually do. So, at the next session, I said to her, "Can we talk about just how we related to each other in the session last time?" And she said, "OK." And I said, "So how did you feel about how we related to each other or I related to you?" And she said, "Well, it was OK."
>
> I know she tends to not know how she's feeling, so I said, "The reason I'm asking is I felt I pushed you a lot harder and tried to get you to do things in a way that I've never done." She said, "Yeah, you did that." And I said, "Yeah, I thought I did. So how did you feel about that?" She said, "Well, it wasn't so great, but I know I need to do these things." And I said, "But it didn't feel very good, did it?" She said, "No." I said, "Did it make you want to do the things I said?" And she said, "No." I said, "OK, so can we back up a little bit?" She said, "Sure."
>
> When I went in this week, she had put some of the things into practice and she was up a pound. I think it made her feel better, and I know it made me feel better. When I walked out the week before, I knew it didn't feel good. Now I realize it was because I was pushing against resistance. I'm also glad I chose to talk with her about the process of backing off. I can tell our discussion made the work more effective.

Sample Dialog: Asking a Client To Help You Structure a Session

This client was just diagnosed with Polycystic Ovarian Syndrome.

Molly: I understand your doctor has referred you to me because you have Polycystic Ovarian Syndrome.

Joan: Yes. And I couldn't wait for this appointment. I'm glad you fit me in this week. The doctor didn't really explain PCOS. She said it might mean I will have trouble getting pregnant and might get diabetes someday. My cousin has it, but she has hair on her face and I don't, so I don't understand. And I read that I have to eat like a diabetic and have to lose weight, but I've tried for years and I just can't. And she said I need to take a diabetes drug, but I don't have diabetes. How do I have to eat to take care of this? Someone at work said I shouldn't use artificial sweeteners, 'cause they make it worse.

Molly: Wow! You have all sorts of wonderful and important questions. I have answers for all of them. I want to help you in the best way I can, and we will not have time to get to all of them today since I only had a half-hour opening. What is most important for you to walk away with today? We could cover the most important issues and then get together again in a week or so to continue.

Joan: Well, the doctor did say that it's not as if I'm going to die from this, so I can take my time figuring out how to eat. What I need right now is to understand this better. It's so confusing. How did I get it? Is it because I haven't controlled my weight?

Molly: I hear that you are wondering if you have brought this on yourself. If I describe more about PCOS and what causes it, would that be what you need?

Joan: Yes. I'm losing sleep over it now. If I did anything to make it so I can't have children, I don't know what I'll do.

Molly: I can assure you that you did nothing to bring this on. Would you like a scientific explanation of PCOS or more general information about the condition and what it will mean to you?

Joan: Oh, don't use all those big science words with me. I barely made it through high school because of science class. I just want to know if it's my fault and what I can do about it.

Molly: OK, I promise I'll leave out as much science as I can. Let me know if I get off track and you need me to explain something differently. Then after you've had a chance to get used to the idea of having this condition, we'll get back together to talk about what you can do. So, PCOS is....

Ways To Check In

- Ask your client **what he wants** to address today. This is particularly useful when there is too much to cover in one session.

- Shift gears occasionally in a session and ask the client if you are addressing **what he had hoped for that day.**

- Ask **what kind of information** this client finds most helpful. For example, the science behind the specific diet recommendations, what outcomes the client can expect from making the recommended changes, or specific ideas of what to eat and how much.

- When it's time to get into brain-storming mode, **ask the client to jump in first** with ideas about how to handle the issue at hand. "I have some ideas about this, but I'd like to hear what you have come up with so far."

- When you are about to **jump in with your advice**, ask the client first if this is what he wants from you.

- Ask the client what **role he wants you to take** in the counseling.

- With a long-term client, periodically ask to take part of a session to **review how the process is going.** Go back to the beginning for a reminder of what the client came to you for and ask what is and is not working well. Ask what you do that is most and least helpful.

- If you find yourself **uncomfortable about a pattern** that has developed in your sessions with a particular client, bring it up. For example, you might notice you spend a large part of the session on small talk, or feel you are doing all the talking, or wonder if you add too many examples from your own life. "Can I check in with you about something? I know I use examples from my life in my counseling. Some people find this helpful and some people find it distracting. Can you tell me whether that works for you or whether you would rather I do that less often?"

Practice Steps: Asking Your Client for Direction

1. Think back over your last few contacts with clients. Did you check in with the client at all? How often? What kind of checking in do you already do? What happens when you do?

2. Do you frequently realize at the end of a session that you missed something important? This could be a clue that you missed opportunities to ask for direction. First, forgive yourself, then design a way to practice this skill.

3. Pick one of the techniques listed in the box that you don't do yet and do it as much as possible for a week. Take stock and see what you learned.

My Experiments With Asking Clients for Direction:

What I observe:

_____

_____

_____

_____

How I will experiment:

_____

_____

_____

_____

_____

Tip #5
How to Respond to Your Client's Strong Feelings

Serenity is not freedom from the storm, but peace amid the storm.

What do you do when your client experiences a strong emotion in your session? What is your role as a nutritionist and what is the role of a therapist? How can you take care of yourself around such strong feelings?

Some basics about emotions:

It may help to remember that there are four basic types of emotions. They can be categorized as mad, afraid, glad and sad (use the mnemonic **MAGS** to remember them). Within each category, these emotions can be expressed in a broad range. For example, afraid can feel as mild as hesitant or as strong as terrified. Mad can be annoyed at one time and enraged or bitter at another.

Shame (the profound feeling of negative self-worth that in its mildest form is embarrassment) is a special case. Some therapists think it is in the sad category while others think it is a unique emotional response.

It is not unusual for one feeling to come out looking a lot like another one. For example, many people (often men) who are feeling vulnerable and scared will act angry. What presents as anxiety can be almost any feeling underneath.

Feelings, thoughts and behaviors:

Feelings are not chosen, controlled or stopped. They simply arise. For example, when we lose something or someone beloved, we feel sad. When we believe we are in danger, we feel afraid. Our *thoughts,* on the other hand, just arise, but we can choose to stop them, direct them or add new ones. Our *behaviors,* and what we say, we can choose.

So of the three, **feelings simply are.**   They can provide useful information but not be forced to change.   There is no such thing as a feeling that is either valid or invalid. If it is felt, it is valid. The *behavior* that follows may be wise, stupid, abusive, immoral, self-destructive, etc., but that's another issue.

If you notice a persistent pattern, refer:

Any client who regularly expresses strong emotion in your sessions would benefit from being in therapy. If he isn't seeing a therapist, this needs to be addressed with the client.

If the client is in therapy, it may help you to bring this pattern up with his therapist. **Ask for guidance** about how best to handle these moments with this particular client. It may be helpful to ask the therapist if this client primarily needs to get better at containing emotions or expressing them, or both. Don't forget that you are required to obtain a signed release before speaking to anyone about your client.

Containing emotion:

Some clients have minimal skills at containing feelings and therefore have trouble functioning in the world. This may be one of the goals of their therapy. Many clients with Post Traumatic Stress Disorder or who experienced early significant trauma, abuse or neglect may be in this category. These clients **can feel scary to be around** at times.

If it feels as if the expression of feeling you are observing is **out of proportion to the stimulus,** it very well might be. It is likely that the present situation is triggering memories that greatly intensify the reaction. It's not your job to help the client make the connection between the present stimulus and the past memory.   If the client is already aware of the connection and you have good rapport, a gentle reminder from you might be in order.

Remind yourself and the client that to work on the nutrition goals you have agreed on, it will be necessary to contain the expression of feelings, valid as they are, to a small portion of the session. **Ask the client to tell you** how it is best for you to respond. One of my very anxious clients taught me to remind him to take a moment to breathe deeply. With another, I have learned that when she cries, if I acknowledge the tears ("This is really hard, isn't it") and sigh with her for a moment, she will be ready to refocus on the food work.

Expressing emotion:

Other clients are working to express feelings more. This is a big generalization, but many of these clients are depressed. When one of these clients shares a deep, true feeling, it is a **precious thing,** and it is appropriate to respond as one human to another with empathy and/or validation. "I can see you are deeply sad about this, Peggy. That's great that you can sit with this feeling and share it with me." You may be in a position to play a valuable role for your client by allowing the expression of emotion when it appears, validating and accepting it.

However, that is **not the *primary focus*** of your work as a nutritionist. With my nutrition clients who see someone else for therapy, I have learned to listen with empathy and then gently remind them with a smile that "yes, strong feelings sure do come up around food." I go on to say how wonderful it is that we have this "window" through food work to these important feelings that they can bring up at their next therapy session. Again, consultation with your clients' therapists can be valuable. Ask, specifically, what they believe you can do to most help the client when strong emotion emerges.

Responding rather than reacting:

There's a difference between having a normal human response to your client's feelings (for example, empathy for her grief, identification with her anger at injustice) and **reacting with your own feelings.** Examples include fear when your client yells or guilt when she says, "This just isn't working." These are some of the hardest moments in sessions. There are short-term strategies to apply and longer-term learning opportunities to take advantage of.

Here's one strategy that helps me: **Stay focused on the client's feelings** as expressed, mirror them back and then ask what she wants to do next. For example, "You are very frustrated, aren't you. You've been eating in an attuned way for weeks and your weight has not gone down. What would you like from me right now?" If you sense that the client is also angry at you, stay curious. "You sound angry. Are you most angry at me, at your body..."

After a session in which you found yourself reacting rather than responding, you can take a deep breath and say to yourself, "Boy, that's an opportunity for learning for me! How can I best explore this?" Other options include writing in your journal, talking with a colleague or your therapist, or bringing it up in supervision.

Your role:

So what is your role as you sit in the room with an **anguished client?** First, distinguish between your role (guiding your client toward health behavior changes while remaining respectful and empathetic) and the therapist's role (may include working on emotion management skills and learning to label and use the information that feelings present).

Simply sitting with a client who is expressing strong emotion, without trying to change the feeling or convince her it's wrong, can have a profound therapeutic effect. Remaining calm and not taking on your client's affect or anxiety has value in itself. Given the opportunity to just sit with an emotion with your client, take it. Then refocus the session on what you remember as the client's goals.

A few words about taking care of yourself:

Even when your clients don't experience strong emotions, nutrition counseling is hard work and takes a toll. Find ways to routinely **nourish yourself.** Regular exercise and yoga help. Even a moment of deep breathing or stretching between sessions can allow the release of affect you may have picked up from one client and reground you for the next one. Find a colleague who is willing to hear you out when you just need to vent or to get a hug. Keep a copy of the serenity prayer handy:

God grant me the serenity to accept the things I cannot change, the courage to change the things I can and the wisdom to know the difference.

This is a complex and very important topic. I've only scratched the surface.

Case Study: When a Client Falls Apart

A dietitian who attended one of my workshops shared this incident on our conference call a month later.

> Nancy: I bring a lot of stuff out in people, and sometimes it gets a little too much. The other day it felt like it went over a boundary. I had to calm my client down because he was so worked up that I was scared. I had seen him about three or four times. I didn't realize there were a couple of incidents in his life that were very upsetting. When he told me, my reaction was, "Wow, is there someone you can talk to about that?" He knows therapy could be helpful but wants to get on with his life. He is also someone who doesn't want me to write things down. He is very concerned about confidentiality. I realized that we needed to save what came up because I'm not qualified to go further.

> Molly: So you wanted to note this is a big deal and help him contain it so he could still function in the world.

> Nancy: Right.

> Molly: How to help clients stay grounded when this kind of thing happens is an important skill. You're not a therapist and you're not trained to do that.

> Nancy: I think the patient needed me to stay grounded.

> Molly: That's, of course, the first step.

> Nancy: It was very upsetting to me. I was worried that I had stepped outside my defined role. Particularly when he said, "You can't tell anybody what we were talking about."

Molly: Did you see any reason not to maintain confidentiality?

Nancy: No, he didn't say he was going to harm himself.

Molly: Good. Remember, being there in the room when someone falls apart doesn't mean you made him fall apart. And also it doesn't mean that you're supposed to be treating him for that. This is someone with a lot of unresolved trauma. You don't happen to do that work – that isn't your job. You are in a position to point out to him that the fact that he can get triggered so easily may make it difficult or maybe even impossible for you to get very far with nutrition. When he's grounded again, you could ask to open a conversation about how you two will work together. You may need to discuss how to avoid triggering his trauma memories. If that seems impossible, you may need to bring up whether he is ready to be working on his eating. Do you feel OK about having that kind of conversation?

Nancy: Well, yes. Can you suggest some language?

Molly: First, establish that he wants to work with you, then request to back up and discuss what happened in the last session. After emphasizing about how scary it may have been, ask if it happens frequently. Ask if he has thought about working with a therapist. If he will not see a therapist, Nancy, you might want to consider whether you're willing to continue to work with him. I gather this isn't someone with a classic eating disorder?

Nancy: Well, that's part of the problem. He definitely has disordered eating associated with traumatic events in his early life.

Molly: So if he did have clear symptoms of anorexia or bulimia, you would say, "I'm not going to work with you without your seeing a therapist. The standard of care is to work with a team."

Nancy: Absolutely, I am used to saying that when I need to.

Molly: It may have taken a little longer for you to pick up on this because it isn't a classic eating disorder.

Nancy: And I see that in some of my obese patients. They may or may not get triggered to fall apart, but it's more like we're having trouble getting anywhere because there are so many issues that get in the way. He's another step beyond that because of the trauma history.

Molly: You are not in a position to diagnose Post Traumatic Stress Disorder, and I wouldn't use that term with him unless he brings it up. You could use more generic terms. "Boy, this stuff in your past can really trigger you and throw you off, can't it?" If he agrees, then you can bring up what you know to be true, that "we're going to need a team in order to help you."

You're talking about the flashbacks of PTSD when he is being triggered to fall apart. In this situation, whether he already has a therapist or not, in order to continue to work with him it's going to make sense for you – the two of you – to have safety edges. This would be a process for catching it when something like that is beginning to happen and to get regrounded. There's absolutely no reason, even if you were a therapist, to allow him to fall apart. A therapist would first build up the client's ability to handle the triggering and back away from it. Eventually, the client would go to those memories, but not as flashbacks. I provide this background on trauma work to show you where you fit in. You can be in a position to help him back off and feel safer, but only if you have discussed it ahead and have a plan. This is for both your safety and his. Eventually, after much work in therapy, there may be a time that these memories are available to him as regular memories, as opposed to flashbacks, and you can talk about how they fit into your food work. It is best to leave it up to him to let you know when he is ready.

Nancy: Well, what I did in the session was a tai chi move. I could tell he didn't want to go there and I didn't know how to stop him. I said let's just take a minute and do some body work. So we did a tai chi move and deep breathing for about two minutes, and it helped, and he said thank you.

Molly: What you did was bring him into the present and into his body. That's exactly what it takes. You can do it by saying his name to him. You can also ask him to focus visually on one object. You asked him to move. You asked him to be in his body.

Some therapists ask clients to put their feet solidly on the floor and feel the floor. You thought of a great way to do it.

Nancy: I'm glad that I have a perspective now about triggering and making a plan with clients who have a history of trauma. I can back off, lighten up, and keep him in the moment. I was worried that I was going to be afraid every time I see him that he's going to get triggered again. Now that I have a plan, I feel safer.

Sample Dialog: Grounding

Andi was a client who called me for a consultation. She had struggled with weight her whole life and wanted to come in to see if she wanted to work with me. She came in looking anxious. Her gaze was down, and she had trouble settling down in the chair. In the first few minutes, she began several thoughts that she didn't finish. Here's my recollection of the next several minutes of the session.

Molly: Andi, you seem nervous.

A: Yes, I really don't know if you can help me. It's so hard...

Molly: I can tell it's hard for you. You're sitting here with someone you've just met trying to talk about something that has troubled you for a long time. Would you prefer to spend a few minutes just getting more comfortable here?

A: Good idea. (Takes a deep breath.)

Molly: Oh, that was a nice breath. Breathing is useful. Is that chair OK for you? Would you like to try that one instead?

A: Oh, I guess this is a little low for me. I'll try this. Oh, that's better. It supports my back better.

Molly: Oh, good. I want you to feel supported here. (We both laugh.) It looks like that chair also allows you to have your feet firmly on the floor. Is that good?

A: Yes. I'm feeling a little better now. I just don't know where to start. There's so much.

Molly: Yes, I guess it is easy to overwhelm yourself. Would it help to focus on just what one thing made you decide to call me last week?

A: Yes, it was the visit to my doctor.

In this example, when I realized that Andi was overwhelmed with thoughts and feelings, I used several techniques to encourage her to become calmer and more grounded. First, I mirrored her state, then suggested she become more aware of her physical comfort. I pointed out a deep breath she took in order to encourage that. I was lucky to find an opportunity for humor. Since she had been overwhelmed with so much to say, I then suggested a way to narrow down what she would talk about first.

Grounding Skills for You and Your Clients

Grounding (or centering) activities bring us to the present and to reality (away from fantasy or memory) and to a sense of safety.

Typical activities:

- Attend to breathing, making it slower and deeper.
- Focus on just a few vivid things in the present (i.e., an object, a sound and/or a sensation) and describe them out loud.
- List reassuring thoughts that are true (see below).
- Change posture, moving into a position that is more balanced.
- Take a walk.

Self-statements that may help your clients:

- "I am safe and OK at this very moment."
- "I have several people who care about me."
- "This fear I am feeling is about old stuff that is not happening right now."
- "It is now Monday, June 6th at 7:18 p.m., and I am in your office. I can feel the chair I am sitting on and you are wearing a white shirt."

Self-statements that may help you:

- "I am a competent professional whether this client sees it or not."
- "My client is very upset. That doesn't mean I need to be."
- "This anxiety is about not knowing if my business will succeed. I have paid the rent this month and there is no need to worry right now."
- "I am very puzzled and unsettled about this client, but I don't have to struggle alone. I can call a colleague or get supervision."
- "I know nothing looks as bad when I look back on it the next day."

Practice Steps: Responding to Your Client's Strong Feelings

1. First, ask yourself if this is a problem for you. Have you ever felt helpless as your client cried? Do you worry you will bring out more emotion than can be handled in a nutrition session?
2. Next, think back over a few recent times that were problematic for you. Remember how it began and how you felt and how it eventually ended. Identify what part is hardest for you. Is it that you hold back asking certain questions because you fear deep feelings emerging? Is it that you don't know what to do if they do emerge? Do you feel as if you are hurting the client and need to get him to put away his feelings?
3. If you have difficulty distinguishing what is so hard for you about this issue, you may benefit from professional supervision.
4. If you try to talk a client out of feelings or to move on right away, practice sitting for a few breaths and mirroring what you hear before asking if the client is ready to move on.
5. Remind yourself of your role (page 180).
6. Practice noticing when you feel upset by your client's feelings and find ways to care for yourself with some of the ideas on pages 34 - 35.

My Experiments With Responding to My Client's Strong Feelings

What I observe:

_____

_____

_____

_____

_____

_____

_____

_____

_____

_____

_____

How I will experiment:

_____

_____

_____

_____

_____

_____

_____

_____

_____

_____

_____

Tip #6
Mirroring

Clarity of observation is possible only when we are able to suspend judgment.
Shale Paul

Mirroring, or reflective listening, is repeating what you have heard in your own words until you are sure that you have indeed heard it fully and accurately. It includes asking your clients if they have been heard.

Examples of mirroring with words:

- "What I hear you saying is …"
- "So you feel …"
- "Let me see if I heard you correctly. You…."
- "It sounds like …"
- "You really care about/want … don't you?"
- "Is there more that I've missed …?"

Most of us use mirroring naturally here and there. Radical mirroring is when you **simply stay with the process** of mirroring and hold no other agenda. It means not moving on to solutions or advice. It means continuing with mirroring until the client naturally shifts.

We can also **mirror a client's emotions.** This is done by modulating vocal tone or words or body language to resonate with the client's emotional state. Generally it's best to do this only briefly to gain rapport and then shift back to a helping stance.

Advantages:

Mirroring allows for the most **accurate information exchange.** It effectively checks assumptions. Many times I have been surprised when I assumed I understood the meaning of something to a client and, after mirroring, a completely different (and important) meaning emerged.

By mirroring, you **show empathy and** respect. Think of the best listeners you know. The ones who make you feel cared about and valued. You feel their focus is on you. It is likely they mirror you often. The next time you are with one of these people, notice what they do.

This approach encourages clients to explore and respect **what is true for them.** Have you ever had an insight or come up with a great idea in conversation with someone who was simply acting as a sounding board? Your mirroring helps clients learn what they need to about themselves to attain their goals.

Mirroring reminds you to stay in a stance where the **answers are in the client.** In order to carefully mirror, you need to stay focused on your client with only a secondary focus on your own agenda. It's good training.

Clients who are mirrored will often shift out of a stuck place. Mirroring **slows the process** and contributes to reflection. For a client who stays in a complaining or blaming stance, holding up a verbal mirror can show her something useful if she is ready to see it. It might be that what she is doing isn't working, or that now she has been heard and can move on, or that her husband isn't really to blame. Let her figure out the lesson; all you need do is mirror.

Finally, mirroring is a safe place to go when you don't know what to do next. The next time **you feel clueless or helpless** during a session, take a deep breath and simply mirror what you just heard and keep mirroring until something shifts. If nothing else, it gives you a chance to catch your breath. More likely, though, it will give you something in the client that you can respond to.

Cautions:

Occasionally a client may get annoyed with your mirroring because she wants something else from you at that moment. If you get this feedback, move along with her agenda. However, most of us **use mirroring much less than we could** and err on the side of leaving it too soon. If we let fear of annoying a client cause us to let go too soon, we may miss something useful. It's better to trust the client to indicate when she is ready to move on.

Expert mirroring **takes practice**. Search for times to play with it.

Case Study: Mirroring To Establish Connection

Several years ago, I had a client, Susan, whom I found very frustrating. She would begin each session as if she couldn't wait to tell me all she had been holding in all week. It was difficult to get a word in at all for at least the first half of our time.

The majority of her talk was about her chaotic life, complaints about her job and her family. It did not seem to me that we were spending much time on nutrition. I had pointed this out to her twice, and she seemed to ignore me. I decided to give up trying to accomplish more of what I thought our agenda was and just listen and wait each time for the few minutes she would allow us to talk about food. I found myself getting bored as I waited. I realized I was bored because she was not connecting with me at all. I didn't know whether this was because she really didn't want to talk about food and was holding me off or whether she was simply not good at connecting or perhaps she just needed a chance to "warm up" each time.

I decided to engage with her about whatever topic she brought in, insisting on connecting, but on her topics. I began to mirror what she was saying. At first, it was mostly just a word or two because I couldn't get in anything else between her words. I could feel a shift. She began to look at me as she talked and even ask me questions. I continued to respond to what she wanted to talk about, carefully mirroring back what I was hearing. After a few minutes, she took a good look at me for what felt like the first time and said, "So what should we do today?" I asked her what she would like to do, and she told me of an upcoming eating-out situation she wanted advice on.

After that, I began each of our sessions with careful mirroring, and she began to shift to nutrition topics earlier in the session. I will never know the reason she needed to ramble on, but my gentle insistence on connecting with her allowed a shift to occur.

Sample Dialog: Mirroring As Problem Solving

This portion of a session with a client shows several benefits of mirroring. See if you can spot them.

Ruth (a client with Type 2 diabetes): I'm having a tough time with my blood sugars recently.

Molly: So, your blood sugars have been high this month.

Ruth: Well, not high all the time. A few have, but I always know what caused it. Like last weekend at my parents 50th anniversary party, I decided to go ahead and have some of everything and to have some of the wonderful cake, too. I knew I'd get high values after that, but it's been a few months since I made a choice like that and just decided to let go.

Molly: So, mostly your blood sugars are not going high except once in a while when you choose to let them.

Ruth: Yes, it's more that they go low sometimes and I can't figure out why.

Molly: Oh, so you want help figuring out what is causing these low blood sugars.

Ruth: Yes, I've been trying to notice patterns like you've told me to. It usually happens in the afternoon when I'm at work, and I think it's mostly on the days that we have a lunch meeting.

Molly: So far you've figured out these mystery sugar drops happen in the afternoon and on lunch meeting days.

Ruth: Right, those days I always get in about an hour earlier because I know I won't have much time to get my work done and want to get an early start.

Molly: Oh, you get in earlier those days.

Ruth: Yes. Oh, and I take my insulin earlier, too. Oh, dear, maybe that has something to do with it. Gosh, you are making me realize I do a lot of things differently on those days. I make my morning snack a little smaller so I can have more of the stuff they feed us at the meeting. Then sometimes they have stuff I don't like. You know I'm pretty picky.

Molly: So, you're saying that your usual schedule that mostly allows good blood sugar control is quite disrupted on meeting days. And since you are particular about your food, you sometimes get a little less to eat.

Ruth: Right. When I follow my usual schedule, it's always fine. I can see I need to take a look at my schedule those days and figure out how to get it closer to the other days. I bet I can do that. I could also find out what they are serving. My friend is the one who talks to the food service people. If they are having things I don't like, especially the protein and starch categories, I can bring something. I did bring some of my favorite bread from home once when I heard they were having baked potatoes, which I can't stand.

Sometimes it's this easy to help clients find their own answers; sometimes we need to supply more information. When they have the answers in themselves, a great way to get them out is to mirror what you hear to be true.

Sample Dialog: Mirroring When You Don't Know What to Do

This occurred about three months into treatment with a 16-year-old with anorexia. She had been referred by her doctor after losing 25 pounds in three months. She had regained some of the weight and had connected well with a therapist.

Jesse: I've decided to go out for the track team.

At this point, I felt like a "deer in the headlights" for several reasons. I knew that she had not gained enough weight to make strenuous exercise completely safe and that before treatment, she had been engaging in excessive exercise at a gym. I was also familiar with her high school's track coach. He did not seem to understand eating disorders, pushed the team in grueling workouts, and once told one of my clients with bulimia that she should lose weight. I began with mirroring to **buy myself time to think** and to **convey respect** for her desires to reduce the likelihood that we would get into a resistance argument.

Molly: Oh, so you've decided to go out for track.

Jesse: Yeah, there is a nice group of girls that run track, and so I could hang out with them.

Molly: So, that's part of it, that you could hang out with them.

Jesse: Yeah, I'm excited about it. They are really nice.

Molly: (after a pause) So, I guess my role is to help you figure out how many calories to add for all that exercise.

Jesse: Calories? How many calories?

Molly: Well, let's see... My initial guess would be about 400 to 500 more calories a day. We could adjust it up or down depending on what happens with your weight.

Jesse: Oh.... I didn't think of that part of running track. It's hard enough now eating what I am. I can't add anything.

Molly: Hmmm. So you really want to be a part of that group and you can't see adding the food your body would need. What a dilemma.

Jesse: Yeah, I really want to do it. Are you sure I need that much?

Molly: Yes. What a tough trade-off for you! To get something you really want, you'd have to give up something else. Well, it's your choice.

Jesse: Darn. (after a pause) Oh, maybe they have room for another manager. I know that Jon is a senior and might have to miss some meets this fall when he visits colleges. Maybe I could do that, 'cause all you do is go with the team and keep the stats. Then I wouldn't need to eat more, right?

Molly: Yes, if you aren't training with the team, you could stay at the same calorie level.

Jesse: I think that's what I'll do.

Molly: OK, but I'd be glad to help you increase your calories at any time if you decide to make that decision. It's up to you.

The mirroring at the beginning of this dialog **gave me time** to gather my thoughts. I realized that her doctor would not sign the permission form to let her join the team. This allowed me to relax and offer my expertise while letting her make her own choices.

When I heard her **ambivalence** emerge, I simply mirrored it back to her several times, inviting her to stay with it long enough to see what might shift. She had a better understanding of the high school scene than I did and, fortunately, realized there was an alternative to running track that would still give her what she wanted. By becoming a team manager, she would not have to take more steps in her recovery that she knew she was not ready for.

Practice Steps: Mirroring

1. First, spend a day or so observing your process of mirroring. Notice the difference between mirroring in your head while nodding your head and actually putting into words what you are hearing or seeing. How often do you tend to mirror out loud?
2. Expert mirroring takes practice. Search for times to play with it. Try mirroring your children and/or spouse several times a day for a week and notice the results. In these informal situations, it feels more natural to just mirror once or twice. If you have permission, you could experiment with doing nothing but mirroring for 10 minutes. (This is an exercise that is often suggested to couples by marriage counselors.)

3. Practice with colleagues and friends. Ask them to talk about something of interest to them while you mirror. Do this for at least 10 minutes even if it feels awkward. Afterward, ask them to discuss the process with you.

4. If you already mirror out loud often, find ways to use it deliberately. Look at the list of useful functions for mirroring in this tip and choose a specific type of situation to practice it in.

My Experiments With Mirroring:

What I observe:

_____
_____
_____
_____
_____
_____
_____
_____

How I will experiment:

_____
_____
_____
_____
_____
_____
_____
_____

Tip #7
Assessing Readiness for Change

*When no answer satisfies, and people continue
to act as if they do not understand,
then the wrong question is being asked.*
Peter Block

We know that if clients are not ready to change we cannot make them. How can we acknowledge this truth and still make progress toward their goals?

The **Stages of Change model** has been around for a few decades. It labels the stages that people naturally go through from "precontemplation" through "contemplation" and "preparation" to "action" and "maintenance." Dietitians can work with this model to match counseling techniques to their clients' stage.

The newer approach of **Motivational Interviewing** adds a practical approach to help clients move through the stages, no matter where they are now. Readiness can be seen as being made up of two parts: importance and confidence.

Importance: (Why should I change?) This is the personal values, beliefs and expectations of clients. Exploring this area means figuring out what matters to them about the change. It also means exploring what change(s) they are ready to address (for example, which ones they believe will make a difference).

Questions to elicit importance:

* "How much does this change matter to you on a scale of 1 to 10?"

- "What might have to be different for the importance to go up a few points?"
- "What matters *most* to you about this?"
- "Are there parts of this that mean more to you than others?"
- "Would it help to talk more about that part?"
- "What specific changes do you believe will most likely get you to your desired goal?"
- "What are the best and worst things about how things are now?"
- "If you were to make this change, what would your life be like?"

The **mind-set** I use when exploring importance is: I don't have a clue what all this means to my client. If I stay curious to find out more, I thereby help the client clarify it too. Then we can work together to move somewhere different. For more detail on how to do this work, see Tip # 20.

Confidence: (How will I change?) This is the clients' belief that change is possible. It is also called self-efficacy.

Questions to explore confidence:

- "How confident are you that you can do this new behavior on a scale of 1 to 10?"
- "What would make you more confident about making this change?"
- "How can I help you succeed?"
- "What has been helpful in the past when you successfully made a change?"
- "What can you learn from previous attempts that didn't work?"
- "Whom can you look to for support?"
- "If we break this change down into smaller pieces, would your confidence increase?"

You can explore confidence about the **overall change** (weight loss or blood sugar control, for example), or you can break it down and explore confidence to do **specific behaviors** (testing blood sugar every morning, walking at lunch two days a week, or decreasing binges in the evening). I find that focusing on confidence to change specific behaviors moves the change process along most effectively. You will gain flexibility as you experiment with various ways to approach confidence with your clients.

Exploring importance and confidence is essential at the beginning of work with clients, but circling back to them from time to time can be helpful, too. For example, when you sense resistance, it may mean you have misjudged readiness and need to revisit **these questions**.

The **practical part** of exactly what to do to change (which foods to buy, how to count the carbs in a bagel, etc.) will come up naturally when you explore what clients need from you. By asking about importance and confidence before launching into the education work, you use the session more efficiently.

I highly recommend <u>Health Behavior Change: A Guide for Practitioners</u> by Rollnick, Mason and Butler for more ideas on applying motivational interviewing techniques in your work.

Case Study: Assessing Readiness for Change

Mary Jane Detroyer, MS, RD, CDN, of New York City, shared this experience that occurred a few weeks after she attended my Counseling Intensive.

> I was counseling a 22-year-old client who had an elevated total cholesterol as an adolescent. I decided to use the techniques from the workshop. He had not gone for a follow-up cholesterol test as he had said he would three months before. I asked him, on the scale of 1-10, how important his cholesterol number was to him.   He said, "Maybe a 6." He saw no reason for it to be important because he was so young. He also said he really didn't know what the numbers meant. I was surprised. I had assumed he knew the connection between blood cholesterol and risk for cardiac disease, particularly in those so young.   I asked if he would like me to explain what we know about the progression of heart disease. After the discussion, he raised his cholesterol number's importance to "11."
>
> I also asked him to rate his confidence that he would get further testing.   At the beginning of the session, he didn't give me a number, but it sounded very low.   As he was leaving, he told me he would definitely get his lipid profile done and wanted to come back to discuss it and work on some diet changes. It was the most amazing thing to experience. Just by focusing my attention on the importance and confidence questions, we got so much further than we had in previous sessions.

Sample Dialog: Working With Confidence to Change

Notice that in this section of a session, we are working on a concrete, behavioral change. The client believes this change will move her toward her family's goal of helping her 6-year-old son's weight move back toward his normal growth curve.

Amy: You are right. Andy drinks an awful lot of soda and juice. I'll bet he will lose weight if I take that away.

Molly: Let me remind you that the doctor does not want him to lose weight, but to instead eat in such a way that his weight will likely drift back to where he was on the growth curve until two years ago.

Amy: Right, that's what I meant. I know we started having more soda in the house since I married Joe. He loves soda and has to have it around.

Molly: Well, let's see, what is your confidence right now on a scale of 1 to 10 that you could go home and set up your house so that Andy would drink less soda and juice?

Amy: Oh, about 3 or 4.

Molly: What makes it 3 or 4 instead of 1?

Amy: Well, I could stop buying the juice. It's really not real juice anyway, and neither Joe or I like it. It's just for Andy. So, I'll just not get more. And I know he likes to drink out of his water bottle with the action figures on it, so we could get some more of those and keep them in the fridge.

Molly: Great idea, Amy. What makes your confidence 4 instead of 7 or 8?

Amy: I'm afraid he will throw a tantrum.

Molly: Oh. So he sometimes does that when he doesn't get what he wants? Are you worried you will just give in and give him some soda or juice to keep him quiet?

Amy: Yes, especially if it's late in the day. I'm tired, and it's so hard.

Molly: I'll bet it is. Are there other times he begins a tantrum about something you know is dangerous and you have no problem staying firm?

Amy: Oh, yes. The other day, he wanted to stay in the toy department while I went to the complete other end of the store to look at clothes. I certainly wouldn't let him do that. Not with all those crazy people out there.

Molly: So you stayed your ground. How long did it take for him to calm down?

Amy: Well, let's see. He kept it up as we walked through the store, but then I decided to tell him about our plans for a movie later that day and that distracted him. He wanted to know which one we were going to see.

Molly: That must have been uncomfortable for you at first in the store, but you managed to tolerate his behavior for a few minutes. And you do know how to distract him.

Amy: Yes, I hate it when he yells like that, but when I know I am right, I just focus on that and it does blow over.

Molly: So, do you think you can apply that approach to any tantrums about beverages?

Amy: Yes, now that I know how important it is.

Molly: So, how else can I support you on this change?

Amy: It's not you, it's Joe. I know he's not going to give up soda and that doesn't help.

Molly: Hmmm. Can you talk with him about it?

Amy: Well, I could try. He does love Andy a lot and is worried about his own weight, too. But, I know he loves his soda.

Molly: Well, why don't you start there? Do you think he will understand Ellyn Satter's approach that we talked about, where you two make decisions about what foods to have in the house and to serve and then let Andy decide how much to have?

Amy: You know, if I talk with him about it as a parental responsibility thing, he might get it. Being a parent is new for him and he really wants to do it right. Yeah, that's what I'll do.

Molly: That sounds like a good start. And if any of this doesn't work the way you had hoped, we could take a look again and develop other ideas. You are great at coming up with things to try out. At this point, what number do you think would describe your confidence to do this?

Amy: Oh, at least a 7. I know I can just not buy that awful stuff and I'll remember to hold firm if he has a tantrum and I can distract him. I'll talk to Joe. I don't know how that will go, but I will talk with him and now I feel like I at least know what to say.

Molly: Great. When I see you next month, I'll be curious to hear how it's going.

Practice Steps: Assessing Readiness for Change

1. If exploring and working with importance and confidence are new for you, pick a certain period of time (for example, one week) or one type of client (all the newly diagnosed diabetics). Keep the Questions to Elicit Importance handy and in view as you work with these clients. Throw in some of them with each client. Be sure to ask the scaling question about the overall issue (blood pressure, for example) and also search for opportunities to ask the degree of importance for more specific parts (getting off medication, for example).
2. Observe what happens. Do you learn more about the client and what motivates him? Does he come up with some issues that surprise you or him? What questions seem to work best for? Which ones do you avoid? Consider tossing in those difficult ones anyway and see what happens.

3. After you gain confidence and skill exploring importance, set up an experiment to work with confidence. Keep those questions handy and open up a time to do this with each client.

4. If you primarily use these techniques in initial sessions, begin to integrate them into follow-up sessions, too. One way to get in the habit of this is to review the clients coming in for a day or week and pick a few whom you feel stuck with. Put a sticky note in the charts reminding you to revisit what is important to them and to explore their confidence to make specific changes.

My Experiments With Assessing Readiness for Change

What I observe:

_____
_____
_____
_____
_____
_____
_____
_____
_____

How I will experiment:

_____
_____
_____
_____
_____
_____
_____
_____
_____

Tip #8
Designing an Environment
to Support Your Work

*Change and growth take place when a person
has risked himself and dares to become
involved with experimenting with his own life.*
Herbert Otto

Asking for support is not weak; it's smart.

Are you satisfied with your life and the quality of your work? No? You're not alone. Most of us, when we're disappointed with our performance or results, blame ourselves and resolve to try again. We figure out how to work harder, study more, stay at work longer. Usually all that gets us is exhaustion.

There is another way:

You can choose to design your life, the people around you, and your whole environment to support your best work. Many aspects of your environment can be altered to better support you. They are tangible and intangible. Here are some to get your creative juices going:

♦ **Workspace:** What is important to you? Quiet, clean, comfortable chair, natural light, pleasing colors and design…. What do you need on hand? Food, fresh water, reference books, easy access to client records….

- **Time/schedule:**   Amount of structured vs. unstructured time, clients scheduled at times of day you do your best work, blocks of time for replenishment, concrete deadlines (or not), vacations (what kind and how long)....

- **Home:**   size, location, colors, light, comfort of furniture and bed, design/style, order/clutter....

- **Outdoors/nature:**   What kind do you respond to?   Water, mountains, gardens....

- **Body:** Our body is our most important environment; it's always there. What can you do to care for it so that it supports you in ways that matter?   Yoga, weight training, cardiovascular workout, addressing health issues, those exercises the physical therapist gave you that help when you do them.   Then, of course, there is the obvious one: food. What do you know about how to feed yourself to be at your best?

- **Values/beliefs/thoughts:**   Have you questioned the values you have had for years to make sure they still work for you?   Are your daily thoughts and underlying beliefs about people and the world supporting you? Examine your routine thoughts, the internal soundtrack you live with.   Does it contain negative self-judgments?   These drain you and keep you stuck rather than pulling you forward. Find the thoughts that nurture and propel you and choose to focus on them.

- **Knowledge:**   Do you need to research some things?   What regular knowledge is useful for you (knowing the weather report) and what might not be (knowing your weight every day)? Do you have ready access to a colleague or supervisor who can give you the kind of advice you need?

- **Possessions:**   Too many or too few?   Does maintaining them drain you?   Could you get rid of some and gain more space/energy?

- **Resources:** Cash/information. Do you need more cash reserves to feel secure? What level of being connected to information streams (news, e-mail lists) works best for you?   Do you need to limit some?   What news source is best for you? What amount of professional training and reading is ideal?

- **Systems/automation:** What systems do you have for routine chores and for accomplishing broader goals? Would more use of technology remove some stress?

- **Family:** Are these relationships nurturing or draining? Would an investment of time and/or attention here yield more support?

- **Friends:** Enough or too many? What kinds of friends support you best? Do you get enough validation, enough challenge?

- **Colleagues/clients/employees:** Examine your client base. Is it balanced to support you financially and emotionally? Is it time to limit eating-disorder clients and look for clients who provide gratification sooner? What about your colleagues? Do you have enough contact with them if you work alone? Would a regular time to get together support you?

- **Roles:** Do you feel stuck in a certain role in some settings? Could you play with stretching yourself into other roles or letting some go?

- **Standards/boundaries:** When you sense resentment, that's a clue you could use some boundaries.

- **Framework/mind-set:** Notice how your mind-set with a given client can shift your energy level. A classic example is when you notice you are working harder than your client. It is time to back off and let the client take over. (See Tip # 10, Reframing.)

- **Mission/vision/inspiration:** Do you have a vision that pulls you forward? If not, consider working with a coach or spiritual adviser to develop one.

This process is so powerful because it **takes the focus off you and your performance** as the sole source of the problem. It's simply not true that it's all up to you to do better. Why work so hard when life can be more effortless?

This shift in focus can **work for our clients, too,** especially the ones adept at self-flagellation. Helping them find ways to support their goals by redesigning their environment is fun and brings gratifying results. Begin fine-tuning *your* life, and as you get the hang of it, share it with clients, friends and family.

This has just scratched the surface of what you can gain from tweaking your environment.   Play with these ideas, brainstorm with others, or look for a life coach to guide you.

This Tip was inspired by the work of the late Thomas Leonard, a leader in the coaching movement.

Case Study: Tweaking My Life

Through three years of work with my life coach, Cohen, Lorraine , I have learned to shift and adjust many aspects of my environment, leading to profound improvements in my happiness and effectiveness. I love the process, and it has become as much a part of me as breathing. I now see my life as one experiment after another. I learn each day what matters to me (and what doesn't) and apply the lessons as I go.

Here are just a few examples of this tweaking process. Many involve playing with my schedule with an eye to achieving balance and efficiency. When I determine that a certain schedule works, I set it in place as a given, and it becomes part of my supportive environment.

- I know that I enjoy and get the most benefit from exercise in the morning, so two mornings a week I don't schedule any clients until 11 a.m. I have chosen Tuesday and Thursday because these are the days my cycling friends meet for a 30-mile bike ride ending at a coffee shop. During the months that it's too cold, I stick to the schedule and go to the gym.
- I have discovered that I write fastest and best early in the day, so I block out time to write in the morning or early afternoon. This is also the best time for me to work on projects that require creativity or initiative, such as product development and marketing.
- I wait to do tasks that demand less of me later in the afternoon or evening. This includes responding to most e-mails, administrative tasks, and backing up computer files.
- Most of my great ideas come from bouncing ideas around with others. To keep this energy going, I have learned to do several things. I make a point of scheduling lunch with certain resourceful colleagues on a regular basis. I come away with plenty of energy and

ideas that justify the time. I also look for colleagues to plan presentations with rather than doing them alone. When I am stuck on a project, I don't hesitate to reach out to those who have assisted in the past. This way, I have a constantly evolving support team.

♦ Keeping up to date on professional reading is a challenge for me even though I enjoy it. I have learned to bring nothing but journals with me the one day a week I take a train to my downtown office. I am then supported to do this reading on a regular basis.

♦ I know that when I am feeling overwhelmed it is time to find a way to automate, outsource or systematize. Just a few examples in my practice include switching to an automated E-zine system for my Tip series, finding a virtual assistant to handle workshop registrations and handouts, and using Microsoft Outlook files to separate e-mail into categories so I can respond to them at the most efficient times.

♦ I have discovered that I do focused work, such as writing, best if I get at least a 10-minute break every 90 minutes. I have learned to fit this in, even if it's just a walk down the block to the mailbox or reading the newspaper.

♦ One of my most important environments is the thoughts in my head. When it is time to make a decision about anything from taking on a particular client who may be difficult or an important business move, I know I need my thoughts focused on my core values, what matters most to me. Once I remind myself of these values, the decision falls into place.

Most of these changes I have embarked on first as experiments. For example, "I wonder what my life would be like if I did some yoga every single day (either a class or 20 minutes at home)?" I then run the experiment long enough to get answers, apply what makes sense and drop the rest.

I now feel I have tweaked my life to within an inch of perfection (to the extent there is such a thing as perfection). As I shift to new phases, I continue to tweak away.

Practice Steps: Designing Environments

1. Search for the small changes that will yield the most. Close your eyes and run through your usual day. When do the energy dips happen? Who is around, where are you, what are you thinking, what isn't working smoothly?
2. Then ask: What would it take to get more flow at that point? Search for areas where your environment could take care of some details and free you to focus on what you really care about. Whether it's automated bill paying or hiring an assistant, there are ways.
3. Notice the environments or contacts that empower you most. How do they do that? Look for ways to get more.
4. Many aspects of your environment could use some tweaking. You may be amazed at how much benefit you get from minimal change. Start with the small ones: blocking out time for yoga, clearing that pile on your desk, or not scheduling clients during your lunch hour. If you are focused on the big changes, such as leaving a job or moving to a new home, you may miss the little, easy ones you can do now.

My Experiments With Designing My Environment

What I observe:

_____
_____
_____
_____
_____

How I will experiment:

_____
_____
_____
_____
_____

Tip #9
Dealing With Resistance

*Integrity is when what you do, who you are,
what you say, what you feel, and what you
think all come from the same place.*
Madelyn Griffith Haney

Susan Krems, RD, of Denver, asked for ideas on holding clients accountable. This got me thinking. Accountability means a willingness to accept responsibility for one's actions. The old term, still used by many doctors, is compliance. Indeed, it is frustrating when our clients do not appear to accept responsibility for their behavior or do just the opposite of what we know is good for them.

It may be helpful to look at the issue from the perspective of resistance.

What does resistance sound and look like?

"Yes, but…"

"Well, I guess I could try."

The client returns for the next visit and has not done what you thought he had agreed to.

The client does not return for a scheduled visit.

Body language that looks like reluctance.

Resistance is what happens when we expect or push for change when the client is not ready for that change. Resistance is not something that exists in clients in a static sense. It arises as a normal, expected product of the interaction. When resistance emerges, there are good reasons the client is not ready to change in the way we are asking. The reasons may not be clear to us or to the client, but they exist. Ignoring them gets us nowhere.

Ways to lessen the chances of eliciting resistance:

When we **emphasize personal choice and control,** resistance will be minimized.

Examples of promoting choice:

- When you brainstorm with a client who struggles with bulimia other ways to cope with strong emotions, urge her to include binging and purging as **one of the options.** This demonstrates her degree of choice.

- When a client wants to pursue a behavior you do not believe will work or disapprove of, before giving your opinion, begin with: "That is one of **your choices."**

- I often use this approach when clients are berating themselves. I don't believe self-criticism helps at all, but arguing with clients tends to bring up resistance. I begin with, **"You can choose** to call yourself those names and focus on what you dislike about yourself. Does it lead to the results you want? If not, would you be interested in other ways to talk to yourself?"

When addressing the lack of a change you expected, be willing to look at what happened **without judgment:** "Oh, that's interesting! I wonder how that came about."

Our clients' behaviors are indeed much more in their control than in ours, so it makes sense to acknowledge this out loud and get back to what we *can* do to help them reach their goals. Unless they have contracted with you to be their food police and follow them around all day, leave them with the choice and control and stay in a consultant role.

Another important strategy is to **track closely a client's readiness** and check in along the way. (See Tip #7.) Carefully exploring how important the change is to her and her confidence in doing it can save time and aggravation later.

Approaching each possible **behavior change as an experiment** (see Tip #3) can lessen the chance that resistance will emerge. When you take that approach, clients are only accountable to you to run the experiment. You are not asking them to commit to the change forever.

How to respond once resistance surfaces:

The general approach is to **back off and come alongside** your client. The sooner you catch it and respond by backing off, the sooner you and your client can get back to work. As long as you push when resistance is present, the work will get nowhere.

This may sound like:

"I can tell I've gotten us off track here. Can you help me review what is important to you right now?" (Going back to checking on importance and meaning.)

"I agree. There's no point in trying something that's not going to work." (Mirroring client's low confidence to change.)

"I see, you really do hate gyms. Since you would like to be more active, would you like to brainstorm other ideas together?" (Acknowledging the resistance and coming alongside.)

"I sense you aren't ready to work on this right now. That's fine with me. This is your session." (Emphasizing personal choice and control.)

"Thanks for reminding me that we need to do this in ways that will work for you." (Implying choice and control)

Some thoughts about eating disorders:

With eating disorders, **ambivalence about change** is often deeper, and more subconscious than with medical nutrition therapy clients. There may be significant medical consequences of the clients' choices, so we and their families feel a strong temptation to push. Control issues often are a central theme in the psychological picture of an eating disorder. It's clear why resistance can be powerful.

Working with this population demands that we **pay careful attention** to not provoking resistance. No matter what we do, it will still come up. We will be most effective if we clearly acknowledge resistance as soon as it comes up and then work with it. Fighting an eating disorder head-on always leads to failure. Finding ways to come alongside eating-disorder clients is one of the most challenging and gratifying aspects of the work.

When resistance doesn't surface:

There may be a few clients for whom **plain old accountability** really works. These tend to be the clients who are clear about the importance of change, and have confidence. They can easily use input on how to accomplish it. All they need is someone to report to and help with making plans for the next step. After a while, the changes become habit and they end with you. Boy, those clients are great, and every now and then, we get lucky and one walks in.

Case Study: One Dietitian's Progress

Cynthia Rife, RD, from Carlisle, PA, attended my Counseling Intensive. As we were ending, she decided to work on backing off and coming along side a client as soon as she senses resistance. She realized she had been continuing to push with resistant clients and wanted to try something new. When she checked in with me a month later at our follow-up call, she was pleased to report that she hadn't even needed to practice backing off. She had begun to work with clients to more carefully track their readiness and unpack what is important to them. Because she is keeping her own agenda aside and focusing on theirs, her clients have not resisted her. She feels like she is working along side them already. As a result, several clients have moved forward with changes they had resisted for weeks. Cynthia is more effective and enjoying her work more and her clients are feeling more effective too. What a wonderful example of how perfecting our process with clients leads to better results all around!

Language for Working with Resistance

To acknowledge resistance and back off:

You sound reluctant. How about we let that plan go and design one that fits better?

There sure is a part of you that doesn't want to make these changes.

You believe that idea won't work for you.

I see, you really do hate gyms. Since you would like to be more active, would you like to brainstorm other ideas together?

I feel like I'm arguing with you and I don't want to do that. Let's take a step back.

To shift into tracking readiness:

I can tell we've gotten off track here. Can you help me review what is most important to you right now?

I don't want to lose touch with what brought you here. Let's see, it was...

Oh, so you're saying this is something you are not confident you can do? Let's revisit your confidence about this and other changes.

I agree there's no point in planning something that you don't believe you can do. How about we break this down into smaller steps?

To promote client control:

I sense you aren't ready to work on this right now. That's fine with me. This is your session. It needs to work for you.

What do you need from me today?

What would you like to work on next?

I have some ideas about that, would you like to hear them? (before offering advice)

How can I best support you?

Let's review how our work is going. What is working for you and what isn't?

To mirror ambivalence:

So you are someone who...

So on the one hand you... and on the other, you... Is that right?

I'm hearing that you feel two ways about this.

To work with experiments:

This does sound scary for you. Maybe we could design an experiment together to gather more information about all this.
We don't know what will come from this experiment. Are you willing to run it just for this week, keeping an open mind and staying curious?

Let's see, what kind of data would be useful to look for? Are you curious what will happen?

No matter what happens, *something* about it will be useful.

I hear that you are not sure you can do this even once. Let's just pretend you are going to run this experiment. How would you set it up? What would you do first? What do you imagine would happen?

Sample Dialog: Backing Off When Resistance Appears

This client is a 16-year-old who gained a few pounds over summer vacation and decided to go on a diet. She liked the attention she received after losing 10 pounds and continued to diet. She became progressively more restrictive with her food variety and was eating a very small range of low-fat foods. She was referred for treatment after losing 25 pounds and losing her period. This is the third visit. At the previous session we had talked about her frustration at not being able to eat with her friends since they ate a broader range of foods. I had hoped this would provide motivation to add back some foods. In the first section of this dialog, I am pushing for change and Jesse is politely resisting.

Molly: So, Jesse, how's it going this week?

Jesse: It's been fine.

Molly: I was looking at your food records and I can see that you are eating the same things day after day. I know we talked about adding foods, more variety so you could eat out with your friends. You seem to be eating the same stuff.

Jesse: I need to be healthy and I like this way of eating, and I can still go out with my friends and just not eat those junky foods they eat.

Molly: So it wasn't a motivation to add back some foods to eat with your friends?

Jesse: I think I can balance the two. I can still hang out with them.

Molly: Well, we also need to figure out how you are going to get a little more calories and protein in because you are still not getting enough. And I know the doctor is really worried about that. Do you think you could get more of what you are eating now?

Jesse: I think I'm doing well now. I'm exercising, I have energy. I feel healthy and good about myself.

Molly: The other thing we are worried about is your bones, especially since your weight is low enough that your periods have stopped and you are not getting enough calcium. We're worried you will get osteoporosis when you get older.

Jess: I know my mom keeps talking about that; my grandmother has it. But, I just feel like I'm strong. I'm doing well. I feel healthy for once.

In this second section of the session, I back off, acknowledge the resistance process and ask her to help us find a way to move forward.

Molly: (shifting back in my chair and putting down my pen) You know, Jesse, this arguing isn't getting us anywhere, is it? We're just going back and forth. Let's see if we can find a way to look at it differently.

Jesse: You're right.

Molly: (speaking more slowly than in the first section) Jesse, could you do me a favor and remind me of something? When you first came in here a few weeks ago, what did you want from me? What was the main thing you wanted to accomplish?

Jesse: The main thing was to get my mom and the doctors to stop hassling me about this protein and my weight. I want it to all go away.

Molly: Right. Thank you for reminding me. You're absolutely right. You were sick of them bugging you. And your mom isn't letting up, is she?

Jesse: No.

Molly: This is frustrating for you. So, let's see, how can I help you with that goal? Hmmm.

Jesse: You could be on my side and try to help me because you are a nutritionist. They'll listen to you. You can help get them off my back.

Molly: I'll bet you are right that they will listen to me more than they will listen to you. And I'd be glad to do that. I'd be glad to tell them that you can stop seeing me, that I "graduate" you. As soon as you are getting enough protein and we see that your weight is OK, I'd be glad to. I'll even write a letter to the doctor.

Jesse: Great.

Molly: Let's see…. How are we going to do this? How can I help you, especially with the protein issue?

Jesse: Well, I'll eat more protein; I just don't want the calories and fat involved.

Molly: So, if we talk about which foods have a lot of protein but are lower in calories and fat? That would be helpful for you?

Jesse: Yes.

Molly: OK. Let's do that, and let's see…. How much protein are we aiming for?

Jesse: Well, you told me 60 grams, and I looked it up on a diet Web site, and it calculated 60 grams for me, so I know that's how much I need.

Molly: (picking up the food records sheet again) OK, let's look at the foods you are eating now that have protein in them and start from there.

Jesse: OK.

What Makes Backing Off So Difficult?

It is easy for us to fall into the trap of continuing to push even when we know the client is resisting. How does this happen and what can we do?

We are acutely **aware of the consequences** of the client's behavior. For example, working in a diabetes program you may see those who have had poorly controlled blood sugar for many years and have developed serious complications. You may have come to care for your newly diagnosed clients and wish for them a long, healthy life. Remind yourself of your role (education and guidance for behavior change) and your clients' role (living life on their own terms).

You may pick up a client's (or family member's) urgency ("I have to lose weight," "Make him stop eating like that") or anxiety ("It's too scary"). You will naturally ally yourself with that side and thereby provoke resistance. **Taking on the concerns** and energy of clients is common, but it doesn't aid the process of change. By backing off, we provide a "holding environment" that allows for ambivalence and a true conversation to occur that may lead to lasting change.

It **feels great to be successful.** Our desire to see clients change quickly can easily cause us to push them. Sometimes part of being a professional is to hold back getting our needs met in the relationship. Holding back your wish for positive results can allow the client enough room to shift.

You may experience **pressure for change and "results"** from other treatment team members. Share with others on the team your assessment of the client's readiness for change. This shifts the focus from blame to a neutral understanding of what is true.

Practice Steps: Dealing With Resistance

1. Search for times you pick up resistance in your sessions. First, just notice it. Make a mental note of how you know resistance is occurring. Is it visual (body language)? Is it a tone of voice? Is it direct, negative words or phrases? Is it a feeling in you?

2. As you are ready, begin to acknowledge the resistance out loud. Choose "I" and "We" statements from the lists in this chapter.

Notice what happens in the session when you stop to acknowledge what is happening.

3. Eventually, add to your repertoire the other steps such as tracking readiness, offering choice, and suggesting experiments.

4. We all continue to push at times when a client is resisting. Make a note of these times in your sessions. Consult the list in "What Makes Backing Off So Difficult?" and pick out which traps tend to catch you. Look for support either through supervision or talking with a colleague.

My Experiments With Dealing With Resistance

What I observe:

_____
_____
_____
_____
_____
_____
_____
_____
_____
_____
_____

How I will experiment:

_____
_____
_____
_____
_____
_____
_____
_____
_____
_____

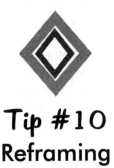

Tip #10
Reframing

Everywhere is walking distance
if you have the time
Steven Wright

Our clients get stuck in ways of perceiving themselves and their world that won't allow change. A reframe can help shift them out of a stuck place. Reframing a problem involves placing it in **a different context** (or frame) and thereby changing its meaning. In our work, this often means taking something seen as bad (a problem) and shifting either its content or its context so it can be seen it as useful rather than bad. The new perspective leads either to acceptance or to creativity about what to do differently.

Examples in nutrition work:

♦ A client is frustrated at slow or no weight loss for months: This may represent the first time in years that her weight is stable instead of always going either up or down. That's progress! Feeding herself daily without either dieting or being out of control is an achievement worth celebrating.

♦ Reframing expected outcomes can be powerful. Many of our clients refer to weight loss as the only outcome they want. This may sound like: "I need quick results," or "I'm not getting the results I want." Framing all their life problems as being about weight keeps them stuck. This is common with eating-disorder clients as well as weight-control or medical clients. To gain some elbow room in their rigid frame, explore what they imagine the weight loss will give them. It may be "confidence," "feeling better about myself," or "a sense of control." **Expanding the "outcomes frame"** to

69

include these larger goals can lead to addressing these goals in other ways while continuing to work on weight loss.

- A bulimic who is struggling to not purge comes in saying she "failed last night" because after an hour of trying lots of alternate behaviors she purged. In her "black and white" world, she failed because she purged. In a **"progress, not perfection"** frame, she practiced some new behaviors and found out which ones show promise to lessen anxiety.

- Clients often come in saying they are "self-destructive." Their frame allows them to see only how harmful their behaviors are. There is **always some positive reason** to continue the behaviors. Your client could thank herself for the attempt at self-care the behavior represents (short-sighted as it might be). She could remain curious for a few weeks about what she is attempting to do by eating beyond fullness at dinner, for example. Maintaining the frame of "everything is an attempt at getting my needs met" allows her to find other ways to care for herself.

Some thoughts about reframing:

A clue that a reframe may be useful: When clients are stuck in a rigid mind-set or are going around and around with the same story. Chances are **they have no idea that a choice of perspectives exists**. This potential for a larger view is one of the values you can offer.

Play with language that shifts you and your client to a different level:

"You could look at it that way. Would you be interested in considering other ways to see this situation?"
"I guess you still need those behaviors in order to feel safe."
"Oh, so that is how you see it now. That's interesting. I see it differently."
"I wonder if this perspective is the most useful one here."

When a client is stuck inside a particular view, she can't see any other way of looking at a behavior. Often, as the dietitian, we are the ones who introduce a larger perspective. The process always **starts with taking a few steps back**. Encourage the client to look at the situation from 6,000 feet up in a plane or from a "fly on the wall" place.

It takes **a creative state of mind** to generate reframes. It's the same loose, open state that works for brainstorming. This state is completely different from the stuck state. Clients may feel shocked at first to hear a reframe from you, and it may take a bit of encouragement for them to get into a more open state. Encourage them to **acknowledge gratitude** as a short cut to a new frame. For example, too much tempting food can be looked at as a good thing if compared to not having enough food.

If they like a particular reframe, it's wise to **write it down** for future reference. Chances are they will slip back into the old, familiar frame. I keep 3 X 5 cards handy and encourage clients to write down the ones they find useful. It's normal to need help to shift to a new frame many times before it becomes second nature.

Stay in rapport with your clients. When you see an opportunity for a reframe, say so and ask if they are interested in hearing it from you. We can only offer reframes; **it is counterproductive to force them.** For it to be useful, the reframe needs to feel at least somewhat true to the client. Some may be ready to stretch into a frame they would like to believe but don't yet. The phrase "Fake it until you make it" can help. For example, a client of mine decided to live as if she believed she was a worthy person at her current weight, though she had to struggle to do this at first. The important point is that *she chose* to take on this challenge; I didn't force her.

Reframing in supervision:

When you are feeling stuck, ask your supervisor or peers to help you see the bigger picture. For example, you can't see that your client is simply in a necessary stage that may take awhile. Your patience can be the valuable support needed to allow a natural progression. Supervision is the perfect place to get validation that you are still providing value for clients, even when no change is happening.

It's easy to get mired with a client in her limited view. In supervision, ask for help **finding reframes to offer.** Others can go with you to 6,000 feet to see the bigger picture that you may not be able to see when sitting in the session.

Case Study: Reframing in Supervision

In my phone supervision groups, I ask what the members need that particular day. Usually a few will have a case they want help with and that provides the content for the call. Occasionally, one will ask for more general help about a particular topic or stuck place. On one call, Anne complained that she was burned out and wondered if she should give up her practice. She had begun her private practice about three years before and was successful and loved it. She complained of being low on energy and caring less about her clients. These are indeed signs of possible burnout. We explored what had shifted in the last month or so. Anne shared that she was 10 weeks pregnant with her first child. She was greeted with immediate and unanimous responses from those of us on the call who are already mothers. We had all shared her experience of being exhausted and of shifting priorities away from what had once been engaging for us. We told her stories that included taking naps on a desk and daydreaming during client sessions. We could hear Anne sigh with relief. As we wound up that portion of the call, she said she realized she was not "burned out," she was simply pregnant. This reframe helped her make the necessary adjustments in this phase of her life.

Case Study: Reframing in Weight Management

Sometimes reframing is not a simple picture or word, it's a whole story the client tells herself. What different, more useful story is there? My client Jodi took several sessions to tell me the saga of her struggle to weigh less. The title of the story was "The One Big Failure in My Life." During the course of our work together, she reworked the story to include the times she had been told by family members and the culture that her body was too big. Looking back, she saw that she was not fat, just bigger than many of her peers. She began to accept that she is a large woman and that, of course, she "failed" at trying to become something she wasn't (i.e., small). With sadness, she began to tell the story that she had tried for years to change her very nature. Later versions of the story included the strength and persistence it took to fight to be the big person she is. She is also a big personality, and she wove this into the story. To be small, she would have had to give up the wonderfully large parts of her self. Now her title is "My Big, Beautiful Self," and her favorite quote is from Marianne Williamson: *"Your playing small serves no one."*

Famous Quotes as Reframes

"I have not failed. I've just found 10,000 ways that won't work."
Thomas Alva Edison

"I am always doing that which I can not do, in order that I may learn how to do it."
Pablo Picasso

"The aim of an argument or discussion should not be victory, but progress."
Joseph Joubert

"When we long for life without difficulties, remind us that oaks grow strong in contrary winds, and diamonds are made under pressure."
Peter Marshall

"Life is not holding a good hand; life is playing a poor hand well."
Danish proverb

"Instead of waiting for the perfect opportunity, I should work toward a realization that every opportunity is perfect."
Suzan-Lori Parks

"Tears are often the telescope by which men see far into heaven."
Henry Ward Beecher

"The great advantage of being in a rut is that when one is in a rut, one knows exactly where one is."
Arnold Bennett

"There are two ways to live your life. One is as though nothing is a miracle. The other is as though everything is a miracle."
Albert Einstein

"Happiness is not a destination. It is a method of life."
Burton Hills

Reframes Can Be Fun

Consider gratitude...

For the taxes I pay, because it means that I am employed.

For the mess to clean after a party, because it means that I have been surrounded by friends.

For the clothes that fit a little too snug, because it means I have enough to eat.

For the stupid things the government does, because I have the freedom to complain about it.

For my aching muscles, because I'm strong and am able to work hard.

For the alarm clock ringing much too early, because it tells me I am alive for another day.

For the gutters that need fixing and the windows that need cleaning, because I have a home.

For the lady behind me in church singing off key, because I can hear.

Practice Steps: Gaining Flexibility With Reframing

1. Practice by playing with family, friends or colleagues. Begin with a complaint or other negative thought and turn it around. Reframes can be fun. Experiment with approaching the process with a playful attitude. Some may fall flat, but it's better to generate a few silly ones on the way to the powerful ones than not attempting at all.

2. When you know a reframe would be helpful and feel stuck, don't expect to do it alone. We often need another person to bounce ideas off.

3. Before offering a reframe to a client, ask if the client is interested.

4. Collect reframes that work with many clients. Write them down and add to them as you think of new ones. Read over them occasionally to keep them fresh in your memory.

5. Sometimes a reframe would help *you* in your work. With a colleague, clarify your stuck place and search for ways to see it differently. Collect the ones that support you in your work.

My Experiments With Reframing

What I observe:

_____

_____

_____

_____

_____

_____

_____

_____

_____

_____

_____

_____

_____

_____

How I will experiment:

_____

_____

_____

_____

_____

_____

_____

_____

_____

_____

_____

_____

_____

_____

Tip #11
Professional Supervision

If one is out of touch with oneself,
then one can not touch others.
Anne Morrow Lindbergh

I not only use all the brains I have,
but all I can borrow.
Woodrow Wilson

Supervision is the process of interacting with a professional colleague for the express purpose of improving your work with clients. It can be done in a small group or one-on-one, in person, by phone, or even e-mail. Supervision has long been the norm among psychotherapists. It is used both in training and in a continuing practice. Many consider it unethical to do therapy without some form of supervision.

Examples of things to bring to supervision:

◆ "I don't understand what is going on with this client?" "What stance should I take?" "How can the client best use me as part of the team?" If the client is in therapy, these questions can be best answered by consulting with the therapist. Especially if you see clients with eating disorders, regular collaboration with their therapist and doctor is essential. Beyond this case collaboration, you may also be able to learn more about the bigger psychological picture. For example, the client may be splitting, keeping secrets, or violating boundaries with staff as she does in her family. You could specifically ask the therapist for more time. She might be open to some short-term supervision.   If your client is not in therapy, consulting with a therapist you feel comfortable with may help you understand what is going on.

♦   "I find myself thinking of my own **body and food issues.**" Sorting out how this is affecting your clients is impossible to do alone. You might use a combination of therapy (to work on your relationship with food and your body) and supervision to explore how it affects your work.

♦   "I feel tempted to tell this client a lot about myself (or I already have) and wonder if it is in the service of the client." **Self-disclosure** decisions are best sorted out with someone else.   (See Tip #1.)

♦   "I know the client in another setting. Is it OK to also be her dietitian?" Some **dual relationships** can work out fine, others get sticky. (See Tip #13.)

♦   "Something doesn't feel right in my work with this client, and I'm not sure what it is." **Vague feelings of discomfort** are wonderful clues that there is something for you to learn and/or something you may be approaching in a manner that is not helpful to the client.

♦   "Why do I feel so annoyed (or bored, or angry, or scared or...) with this client?" These reactions are all examples of **countertransference.** Countertransference refers both to your unrealistic, unconsciously motivated reactions that may be related to past experiences and also to reality-based reactions to the present client's behavior. Reality-based reactions can be a source of insight into the client. Talking it over with a supervisor may help you learn something useful about the client. Reactions that are primarily triggered by your past need to be addressed in supervision (or maybe your own therapy) so they will have a minimal effect on the client. (See Tip #16.)

♦   "Did I step over a **boundary?**" You will get an uncomfortable feeling when you've gone over a client's limit or when she steps over yours. This can be anything from telling a client too much about yourself to a client who calls too often. Talk it over to determine what limits to set and how.

♦   "What process are we stuck in and how can I get us out?" Sometimes we get **stuck in the mud** with our clients and need a colleague's help to see the situation from another perspective. When something keeps happening over and over, ask for assistance to look at it with new eyes and learn from it.

♦ **"Can I get better at this?"** Supervision is the ideal setting for improving your counseling skills. A regularly scheduled time can remind you of your on-going learning process. The frustrations and questions you bring up represent your opportunities for growth. It's a perfect forum to stretch yourself and practice new skills.

♦ **"I'm feeling burned out."** Continuing to work when you are burned out is a disservice to your clients and yourself. A supervisor will get curious with you about how to shift the way you work to be less taxing. You will also get support for more self-care.

Various kinds of supervision:

Case conferences function to share information with other professionals treating the same client and coordinate the treatment plan. In an inpatient setting or clinic, this may be regularly scheduled staff meetings. If you are in private practice, it can be periodic phone calls with your client's therapist. This is of limited value for process and countertransference assistance, unless plenty of time is allowed.

A **group of peers** that meets regularly can bring new perspective to a case and provide support and validation. This kind of group will be of limited help with countertransference and information about psychopathology.

Group supervision with a therapist is an ideal setting to improve counseling skills by bringing up the cases that stump you. A therapist who is accustomed to working with a process perspective (most social workers or gestalt therapists, for example) may be the most helpful. You could learn more about the dynamics of any psychiatric diagnoses your clients may have. Countertransference could be addressed here as well.

A brief course of **therapy for yourself** would give you valuable experience from the client's perspective and allow you to work on any of your own body and food issues. Most therapists would also be willing to help you sort through countertransference as it comes up.

When strong feelings come up in a session, it is valuable to have a therapist who knows you well and whom you trust to check in with. If you do not have one, consider contracting with a therapist for periodic consultations to learn more about psychopathology or to discuss cases so you can build a relationship. Then you could call when strong feelings come up. This kind of **"on call" supervision** can be especially useful for experienced nutrition therapists.

Some reminders:

Use your gut to tell you when to call or bring something up. It's telling you something useful. You don't have to know what's going on, just that you need something. As a matter of fact, my most powerful growth experiences in supervision occured when I simply came with my helplessness and was willing to play. You could choose to welcome that clueless feeling as an opportunity. Generally the hardest stuff to bring up is the most important. It's your area for growth. One value to a regularly scheduled supervision time or group is that it encourages you to bring up the hard stuff.

Supervision is essential when:

♦ You work with eating disorders. At the very least, **case collaboration** is a standard of care. Since these cases can be so complex, having a supervisor to call when needed is advisable.

♦ You find yourself in a **complicated dual relationship** with a client. This could be anything from a client who is also your student to being asked to see the daughter of friend.

♦ Your **emotional reactions** to a client are strong. This could grow into something that would harm the client (and maybe you) if not addressed.

♦ You have struggled with **food and body issues** that continue to come back. Your willingness to go back into therapy as needed is a reasonable way to address this.

Case Study: Supervision

This case illustrates several important functions of supervision including: sorting out countertranference, learning about psychological processes (in this case, splitting), recognizing and maintaining professional boundaries, avoiding burnout, and supporting coordination with a client's therapist.

Susan (a fictitious name because she prefers to remain anonymous) is an experienced dietitian who has been in private practice for three years. She primarily works with eating disorders and recovery from dieting. One day, in group supervision, Susan brought up a client, Judy, age 26, whom she had seen for three weeks. Judy was just finishing a master's degree in sociology and was considering continuing for a doctorate since she was getting perfect grades. She wanted help normalizing her relationship with food, work that Susan loves to do. Within the first few minutes of the first session, Judy was saying how wonderful Susan was, how she finally had someone who understood and could help her. Susan liked Judy and felt flattered by the praise. The work seemed to be going well, with Judy trying everything Susan suggested. Susan heard from Judy's therapist that Judy was very hopeful and that she thought Susan was "the best!" Judy began to send Susan e-mails (sometimes a few per day). Susan responded with brief e-mails, answering her questions and giving encouragement.

By the time she brought the case to me, Susan was beginning to feel something wasn't right. She did not usually spend so much time with one client and realized that she would grow resentful and burn out soon if it continued. She was also puzzled by Judy's repeated statements that she feared Susan would "give up" on her or "leave" her. Susan has never given up on a client. At the last session, Judy had told Susan about her older sister dying when Judy was 9 and having lost several other relatives in the last few years.

First we explored what this client represented to Susan. She realized that Judy's praise felt particularly valuable at this time in her life. Susan was not feeling appreciated in her marriage. Judy's praise felt wonderful, and Susan had been "hooked" into responding to Judy's e-mails with less professional boundaries than she usually would. Susan also was feeling vulnerable to being left by her husband and so had responded to Judy's abandonment fears by overly reassuring her that she would not leave her.

Judy's therapist told Susan that Judy had a tendency to "split" people. Susan was not quite sure what this meant and how it would play out in her work with Judy. I explained that splitting is an unconscious mechanism used by some people to deal with uncomfortable moments in relationships. It involves seeing people as all "good" or all "bad." In extreme cases, the client is unable to hold onto a balanced view of one person and will go from perceiving that person as totally wonderful one day to totally evil the next. As clients, they may perceive one professional as all good and another as all bad. It is more likely that the nutritionist will be the "good" one because the client can talk about food with her but must talk about difficult feelings with the therapist. Splitting is considered a primitive way of functioning used by those who have a poorly developed sense of self.

We discussed ways to minimize the chance that Judy will flip Susan to all "bad" or split Susan and her therapist. Susan's ability to stay consistent in her behavior with Judy is essential, as is setting reasonable and firm limits. Susan will need to stay in contact with Judy's therapist to compare perspectives. As she reviewed Judy's history of losses, she understood the fear of abandonment. It is not Susan's responsibility to help Judy work through those losses; she is responsible only for being there for a steady relationship in which to address Judy's eating behaviors. Susan's first instinct was to respond to Judy's fear of being given up on by responding to every single e-mail and reassuring her very strongly. Ironically, what will serve Judy best in the long run is Susan being consistent with reasonable limits and being quietly reassuring through steady behavior. This might mean not responding to every request. It is likely that Judy's emotional skills are so immature that she will never gain a sense of internal constancy.

Through this discussion, Susan realized that Judy was functioning at a lower level than she had first assumed. Though Judy was achieving academic excellence, her emotional strength was shaky. Susan realized that Judy was going to be a tougher case than she had imagined and that she needed to settle into working with Judy in a manner that she could maintain long-term. Judy will test her over and over, much as a 3-year-old does. Susan knew she could draw on a deep well of patience that has served her through years of child-raising.

Susan left the supervision session with a clearer picture of what was happening within her and getting in the way of the work. She was able to laugh at how her current vulnerability was an interesting (though dysfunctional) fit for Judy's tendencies. Other members of the supervision group sympathized with her home situation and agreed it would be easy to get hooked by such a client. She decided to do more self-care around her personal problems so they will affect her work less. For example, she will plan to spend time with friends who appreciate her and ride her bike more often.

I suggested Susan call the therapist again and tell her how Judy seemed to be idolizing her. She could ask specific questions about how they could best collaborate and what language would be most effective when Judy was feeling insecure. Susan was clearer about her need to set limits with Judy and that this need fit with her professional responsibility. She would talk with Judy about the number of e-mails she is able to respond to per week and work with her to broaden her support network. In the future, Susan will remember to maintain some distance when a client seems to be putting her on a pedestal. Susan decided to bring this case back to supervision off and on for reinforcement and support. She was glad she had stopped to look at the emerging pattern early rather than waiting until her resentment had grown unbearable.

Practice Steps: Using Supervision

1. First ask yourself, what do you need? Is it mostly a more experienced dietitian who can advise you on difficult eating-disorder clients? Are you concerned that your old issues with food and weight will get in the way? Are you feeling lonely in your practice and need support? Do you want to advance your counseling skills?
2. What format do you expect to find most useful? Do you benefit from listening to others' cases? If so, look to form or join a group. Do you prefer to meet in person with a supervisor? Or is a phone session more convenient?

3. To begin your search, you could meet once with each of the therapists you know and respect. Expect to pay their usual therapy rate. A good therapist will be fine with your "shopping around" for the supervisor who will be most useful for you.

4. If you don't know any therapists in your area or don't feel comfortable with any, consider trying phone supervision.

5. Some dietitians may find that a therapist they saw in the past for other issues would be appropriate for a supervisory relationship. Make sure it is someone who has experience with eating issues. You both would need to feel comfortable with and explore this shift of relationship.

6. Another option is to join with a few nutrition colleagues for peer supervision. Unfortunately, these groups can easily slip into informal complaining sessions that will be of little value. It takes discipline to stay on topic. Consider dividing the time so that each of you has a precise number of minutes to present your case or issue and ask for help. You could also search for a therapist whom you would contract with to provide supervision at some of your sessions.

7. Finally, use your intuition to tell you if it is a good fit. After a few sessions, ask yourself if you are getting what you had hoped for. Are you able to bring up *anything?* Ideally, you will feel comfortable enough to bring up even the things that are hardest to admit. Periodically review how it's going. You may find you need to shift to a new supervisor as your practice changes and grows.

My Experiments With Supervision

What I observe:

_____
_____
_____
_____
_____
_____
_____
_____
_____
_____
_____
_____
_____
_____

How I will experiment:

_____
_____
_____
_____
_____
_____
_____
_____
_____
_____
_____
_____
_____
_____
_____
_____
_____

Tip #12
The Power of Acceptance

We cannot change anything until we accept it.
Condemnation does not liberate, it oppresses.
Carl Jung

We can love and accept ourselves and still
work like mad to change ourselves.
Dave Ellis

Our clients come in asking for help with problems. It may be weight they want to lose, foods they eat but know they shouldn't, or diseases they want to avoid or treat. Most of these problems are just that, problems, things they want to get rid of. They may have tried gallantly to combat their problems, and now come to us for help. Our natural inclination is to **take their side against** the problem or behavior.

Trying to stop a behavior doesn't work. When we focus our attention on something, **we attach to it**. The attachment is just as strong whether the focus is on something negative or positive. Our attention causes an attraction much like a magnet. We can fight the pull of a magnet for a while, but eventually we have to let go. We all learned about magnets in grade school. The only way to change the attraction is to turn the magnet around.

Carl Jung and many wise people before him knew what several areas of research are now confirming. In the field of behavior modification, positive reinforcement of desired behavior has proven more effective than punishment of undesired behavior. Janet Polivy and C. Peter Herman's continuing studies of restrained eaters confirm that **fighting unwanted behaviors head-on is ultimately unsuccessful**.

Consider this simple example: Picture a purple elephant in the room with you. Visualize it in vivid detail. Is it a realistic one or maybe made of porcelain and encrusted in jewels? You get to choose. Get a good image of it. Now stop picturing the purple elephant. If the image doesn't disappear right away, focus really hard on not picturing it. What happens? Notice how it is **impossible to not do something**. The only way to stop picturing the elephant is to distract yourself with another image.

This approach is physically manifested in **Asian martial arts** such as aikido and tai chi. A basic teaching is to resist putting your energy into directly confronting an approaching enemy. Instead, students learn to use their bodies to move *with* the momentum of the opponent to deflect the force. Even if you are much weaker than your opponent, by moving in the direction of the momentum, you can prevail.

We have the opportunity as nutrition therapists to show our clients the futility of focusing on the negative and to offer another option. Professionals who fully embrace the **Health At Every Size** Movement naturally work within this acceptance paradigm. It works as well in other settings nutrition therapists find themselves.

Clues that acceptance would be useful:

- You are joining with the client in a head-on fight with a problem behavior.
- You find yourself arguing with a client.
- The client is stuck in self-flagellation about a behavior.
- You are feeling invested in a client changing.
- The client is complaining about cravings or binging.
- You and the client have agreed to take a non-diet approach to weight.

Stances to take:

A classic gestalt therapy approach is **to go *toward* the problem or behavior**. This can include embracing it, getting curious about it, making time for it, or actually increasing it for a time. Accept the impulse behind a behavior while still wishing to decrease the behavior. Monitoring the behavior to learn more about the impulse implies acceptance of it.

Consider **turning toward the problem with curiosity.**   This allows connection with it rather than separation from it. Focusing on it allows teasing apart what it's all about so it can be reworked. For example, with a client who professes to want to record her food intake but isn't doing it, you could say, "Oh, that's interesting! Would you be willing to get curious with me about how that happens?" Chances are your client is berating herself for not recording. Encourage a playful approach that includes simple acceptance that the recording isn't happening and focus on how that comes about.

What about the problem **is worth saving?** The unwanted behavior is so compelling because some essential element has value. You and your client can search for that diamond inside the rock. A common example in eating-disorder work is to explore the process of binging and purging. Many bulimics resist discussing their binge/purge episodes. They want to forget or disown them. Assume the symptom has some useful purpose and gently offer to turn your collective curiosity on that purpose. When the client is ready, she will see the purpose the behavior fulfills and begin to search for other ways to meet her needs. (This work gets very close to the work of therapy, and it is essential to do this in coordination with the client's therapist. Whether you do this work or simply model acceptance of the behavior and suggest she bring it up with her therapist will depend on your skill level and how you and the therapist prefer to work.)

Whenever the client is trying to eradicate something, suggest she **experiment with reserving time** for it, planning it, really doing it carefully. For example, a client of mine had been trying for years to stop afternoon snacking that often felt like a binge. I suggested she work it into her daily schedule, plan what it would be, and make sure not to miss it. I also suggested she remain curious about what made it so compelling.

When a client is really stuck with a repeating pattern, **suggest increasing it.** I know this sounds counterintuitive. Increasing the behavior tends to allow a new perspective on its meaning to the client. For example, with a client who was weighing herself several times a day and was having trouble cutting this back, I suggested she start doing it every half hour. She quickly saw that sometimes she cared more about the number than at other times. She was able to see how she was using it to assess her self-worth when she was feeling anxious. She acknowledged how much it was interfering with her life even at several times a day. It also gave her a reality check about how much her weight naturally fluctuated on any given day. (This is not an appropriate technique with a behavior that has direct and immediate medical consequences.)

This approach to acceptance **applies to** *our* **attitude** as well as the client's. Ironically, when we let go of our investment in the client's changing, we are more able to help her change. It's not easy to let go and get out of the way. This is a perfect skill to work on in supervision. (See Tip #11 for more on supervision.)

This process of acceptance **involves reframing** the situation. (See Tip #10 for more on reframing.)

What if you are willing to go with acceptance and your client isn't?

Model acceptance for the client by suggesting that she could choose to continue the behavior. She's been doing it for quite some time, and it's fine with you if she chooses to continue.

In order to get across the concept that **acceptance is actually more effective than self-hate,** you could remind your client that loving yourself is a necessary first step to taking care of yourself. No lasting change happens out of self-hate.

Many clients are **stuck in self-condemnation** that gets in the way of acceptance and change. Here our first job is to raise awareness. "Is this how you speak to yourself all the time?" "Does it help to yell at yourself that way?" Again, we can model acceptance by saying, "You could choose to continue to berate yourself." And then move on to, "Would you like to explore other ways to look at this?"

Respectfully reflect back that the problem is still there in spite of all the effort to change. Point out that **what they have been trying has not worked.** Are they willing to try something new? (One definition of insanity is doing something over and over the same way and expecting different results.)

Case Study: Acceptance vs. Liking

Sarah, age 47, had come to me to try to lose weight. She had struggled with her weight off and on for most of her life. She said she finally felt ready to address it since her children were grown and therefore she had less stress in her life. As with many longtime dieters, her eating habits were chaotic and restriction-based. She was quickly able to see that this was making it harder for her to eat appropriately. We began to work on eating according to appetite. She picked this up easily and loved the process of listening to her appetite signals and then responding by choosing the food that would hit the spot. Her weight began to drift down.

About two months into this process, her daughter got pregnant unexpectedly and moved up her wedding date. This led to stress in the extended family, who all looked to Sarah for decision-making and advice. Sarah was shocked to notice that her eating became chaotic again and that her weight stopped going down and even began to increase. This is when I began to hear the harsh, critical language Sarah used to berate herself for eating more than she was hungry for. She now had a model for normal eating and had placed it in a position of the "new diet." Since she had "broken the diet," her familiar response was to yell at herself. This led back to a rigid desire to restrict her eating and her usual rebellious response. I could tell we were almost back to where we had started.

Coming from an acceptance approach, I pointed out the significant stress she was under and that she had turned to her usual way to cope, eating. She agreed that this is what was happening but had no other way to respond but to berate herself. We worked for several weeks both on finding her support and new coping mechanisms and on the most useful way to look at what had happened. I felt as if I was beating my head against a brick wall when I invited her to look at her manner of coping with acceptance. I believed that if she could, we could learn more about how her process of turning to food worked so that we could find new ways. I could sense her resistance to approaching the problem this way. Finally, one day I realized that she believed that to accept something meant she had to like it. She clearly did not like the fact that she so easily turned to food when stressed and that it sort of worked. She didn't like it or the results at all and nothing I did or said would change that. I reminded her that accepting and liking are two very different things and shared with her the Dave Ellis quote at the beginning of this Tip.

For months it was still hard for Sarah to see that it was simply true that when her emotions were activated, this trumped her ability to attend to appetite. She wished that were not true. She wanted her feeding process to be completely separated from her emotions. Over time she explored the ways in which her family had unknowingly encouraged her to use food to cope with strong emotions. Again I reminded her that she did not need to like this connection that had been forged long ago, but it was true and accepting it would allow us to find solutions in the present.

Case Study: Childhood Growth Patterns

This case did not end in a satisfying way, and I made several mistakes. It illustrates a common area where lack of acceptance of what is true impedes healthy eating. Terry's parents brought her to me a number of years ago to lose weight. She was a bright, athletic 12-year-old. She had begun to complain about her weight, and so her parents thought she was finally ready to diet. They had wisely not tried to put her on a diet earlier because they thought she was too young. She had always been around the 75th percentile for height and about the 85th percentile for weight. In the last year, her weight had slightly shifted up on the growth chart to the 95th percentile. Her pediatrician had told the parents that, given other physical signs, she would likely start her period soon.

Mom was a petite woman who had a very different body type from her daughter's. I asked about the rest of the family, and Mom told me that Terry looked a lot like her paternal grandmother. She was a big woman who apparently was still proud of having been a successful college athlete. Alone in my office, Terry shared with me some comments she had overheard in school that made her feel she was "too big." She begged me to help her lose weight. I liked her and reacted to her distress by wanting to help her feel better by losing a few pounds (or at least not gain any more for a while).

She liked working with me at first and made a few sensible changes such as decreasing soda and choosing lower-calorie snacks. However, after a few sessions, she got bored with the process and discouraged that she had lost only a little weight. She told her mother she didn't want to go back to see me, and they dropped out. A year later, one of her friends was a client of mine and she mentioned that Terry had gone on several fad diets and often skipped lunch to try to lose weight.

I have reviewed this case many times in the years since. I missed much that was important. First, Terry's slight weight gain just before menarche is normal and should not have been interpreted as a problem. I was not aware at the time that a 12-year-old is not yet completely capable of seeing genetic patterns. It can be the role of her parents, supported by the pediatrician and dietitian, to help her accept the body she has. Terry was right on schedule as an early adolescent in beginning to focus on her body and the changes it was going through. The changes were normal so far, and I could have supported her parents in helping her see and accept her wonderful, strong body rather than trying to make it fit the current cultural ideal. I see now that I picked up what was normal adolescent body anxiety and did not suggest the option of acceptance.

Her mother had apparently long ago accepted that her daughter was a big girl and would always be. This acceptance was unusual and healthy. I lost the opportunity to reinforce this. Apparently Terry's father had not accepted her larger body type and still wished for the petite frame that he so admired in his wife. I don't know how far I could have gotten with this father, but I could have at least spent part of a session exploring what he understood about genetics and what he most wanted for his daughter.

Since seeing Terry, I have stopped myself before being hooked into helping a preteen try to change her body. I insist on carefully exploring what is there to be accepted and celebrated. Sometimes I can help her see her body for what it is and begin the process of acceptance, and sometimes she simply gets angry and leaves. Sometimes parents are relieved to hear their daughter is growing according to her genetic plan, and sometimes they argue with me. But at the least, I offer acceptance as an option.

The Language of Acceptance

For use with clients:

"Oh, so you are someone who loves to bake. ...who hates to sweat ...who finds food comforting at times ...who loses track of your appetite when upset." (Mirroring)

"That's interesting. Does this happen every single time? Would you like me to help you design an experiment to find out more about this pattern that seems to happen so often?" (Encouraging experimentation.)

"How important is it to you to control your blood sugar?" (Unpacking what is important and unimportant.)

"You seem to hope your desire for sweets will just go away. What would happen if you accepted that you like sweets? Might it then be possible to fit them in here and there?" (Pointing out unrealistic expectations.)

"I know you get annoyed at yourself when you decide at the last minute to skip the gym. Does it help you develop the habit of exercise when you beat yourself up about it? I wonder what would happen if you could manage to forgive yourself here and there?" (Reframing)

"I hear how frustrated you are that you still binge every so often. I always assume there is a good reason people turn to food in those moments. Would you like to search with me for what you hope the food will do for you?" (Looking for the positive in negative behaviors.)

To say to yourself about a client:

"I know I cannot make him change. He will either be ready someday or not. I wonder what would happen if I search for his positive characteristics and focus on them instead of focusing on how stubborn he is."

> "I don't like this client's chronic lateness and I never will. What if I just accepted it? Maybe I could make use of the time by reading professional journals or stretching."

Practice Steps: Acceptance

1. Begin with little things. Search for small stuff in your daily life that you don't like, and that you likely can't change. It might be the traffic, the weather, or the slow cashier. Take a deep breath when you encounter these things and remind yourself that it is much easier on you if you simply accept them.

2. A tougher exercise is to search for things in *yourself* that you don't like and haven't been able to change yet or definitely won't be able to. Parts of your body? Your tendency to leave piles of things around the house? The anger that comes up whenever your mother-in-law calls? See what happens when you breathe through your awareness of these.

3. Search for things that your clients have not accepted that you believe are simply true and will not change. Things such as a certain body type, a medical condition, a dislike of exercise, a tendency to turn to food for emotional reasons. Experiment with using the language of acceptance when you notice these.

My Experiments With Acceptance

What I observe:

_____
_____
_____
_____
_____

How I will experiment:

_____
_____
_____
_____
_____

Tip #13
Dual Relationships

Reacting is an emotional reflex.
Response requires thought.
Gail Pursell Elliott

Whenever you have a relationship with your client in addition to the professional one in your office, this is a dual relationships. It might be a neighbor, a friend, someone you run into in the supermarket, your accountant or real estate agent, your lover, or a relative.

Dual relationships can be tricky. They are not necessarily wrong. They do **need to be taken seriously** and examined for potential harm to you or your client.

How might a dual relationship harm the work?

Most people have a natural safety function that acts as a filter when talking about sensitive topics. A clients may consciously or unconsciously withhold embarrassing details if she doesn't feel sure of confidentiality. If there is no dual relationship with you, her internal filter will allow her to be as open as possible. Even if you assure her of confidentiality, the fact that you know her sister or meet at a book group will make it harder to share what might be important to your work. You will likely never be aware of this self-censoring. Your work with this client will just be less effective.

On your side of the relationship, it can be hard to maintain the necessary **professional demeanor**. When chatting with a neighbor we often share confidences equally. In a professional relationship, there is a necessary disparity. It is difficult to make this shift, and it can feel like a loss for you as you appropriately focus on the client's needs. You may

94

also hold back confronting your client about something if the client is also a social acquaintance.

Some guidelines:

Appropriate limits **depend on the type of counseling** you are doing: A goal-oriented client who comes for a few sessions to help get his cholesterol down may be less affected by a dual relationship. When working with eating disorders or weight control, clients may need to reveal deep emotions and painful memories. As a result, they may feel uncomfortable if they see you in another setting.

It is essential to **talk about it** with the client. Don't ignore it! Explore what it is like for each of you, but mostly for the client. Plan to talk about it again after each of you has had a chance to see what effect it has. For example, after the first time you run into your client at your kid's school, bring it up in session. "What was that like for you to run into me?" Is there anything you or your client needs to keep your roles clear?

Many people will initially say, "Fine, no problem." This does not mean that they have thought it through and that your job is done. **Bring it up again**, especially if *you* are feeling uncomfortable.

Be **willing to refer** to another nutrition therapist if you believe it will not be either in your best interest or the client's for you to work with her. The sooner you do this, the easier it will be. For example during an initial phone call you could say, "I have a policy of not seeing people I know already. I'd be glad to recommend another dietitian."

Sometimes it can't be avoided. For example, you are the only nutrition therapist who works with eating disorders within 100 miles. In this case, **it may be possible to set up boundaries.** For example, would it be possible for one of you to withdraw from the other setting in which you meet? Would it help to set limits on what kind of contact would be appropriate? If you avoided all personal talk or food talk when in the social setting, would that be enough? Do you have requests for your client? Does she have any for you? With these necessary, but sticky, relationships, it is best to seek supervision to sort out what you need and what is best for the client.

Use your gut. It can tell you a lot about dual relationships. When asked to work with someone you know, imagine beginning a professional relationship with this person. Then imagine being with her in the other relationship. How does it feel? What comes up for you? Try putting yourself in the client's shoes. How would you feel?

Learn from experiences you have regretted. Look back and ask yourself, "What was the element that made it impossible?" "Was it the depth of work we needed to do?" "Was it the way it ruined my ability to just be myself at the neighborhood picnic?" "Was it that this particular client had trouble maintaining boundaries?" If you have ever been a client in a dual relationship, search your experience for the sticky points.

It's best to **err on the side of caution.** The harm done in a messy dual relationship cannot be reversed. Remember that, just like self-disclosure, it's a bigger deal and potentially more harmful to the client than to you.

Case Study: Dual Relationships

This case comes from a dietitian in private practice who chooses to remain anonymous.

> A person who provides business management services for us and who I have known for a long time, asked me if I would help him with a nutrition program. I knew he could probably afford my fees, I knew that he was motivated and I thought I could help.
>
> And -- there was that little voice inside of me saying, "don't do it." I told him that I had some hesitation about a role conflict and that my clients typically don't know my financial business, but he assured me that he just "wanted a plan". Sigh. I should have stopped there.
>
> So -- against my better judgment I met with him a few times. As it goes with cyclic nutrition enthusiasts, I ended up hearing an earful relative to why the eating was happening, personal issues, marital, etc. I knew very quickly (by the third session) that he needed therapy if he ever had hopes of losing weight permanently. I made the recommendation in that third session. He was a bit taken aback, and then back-pedaled on all the previously detailed problems.
>
> I reiterated that I thought we should make a decision about the dual relationship. In other words, that he be my consultant or I be his, but we shouldn't do both. Unfortunately, it was too late to

make that kind of a break. I was stuck between wanting to keep him on as my advisor and the ethics of acting appropriately with my client. My nutritionist role here demanded that I end seeing him if he was not willing to add the necessary adjunct care.

Eventually he stopped seeing me, saying he would do it on his own. I continued my other relationship with him in the financial arena. The unfortunate outcome is that he didn't get the nutritional care he needed. The waters got too muddy and/or he didn't want to hear the necessity to seek additional services to address the real issues.

Recently he emailed me asking for print or electronic media to count calories. This told me he was still seeking solutions and not wanting to make appointments with me. I offered some advice and felt compelled to offer additional input if necessary. This only partly alleviated my guilt and may have sent a mixed message. We eventually decided to no longer use his business management services.

This case makes me think that if there is a dual relationship, there usually will end up being NO relationship in the end, at least none that is healthy and productive! This is almost embarrassing but I hope that others can learn from this. I have learned that if I am in a professional relationship with someone -- THAT'S IT!! No additional relationships are appropriate. In the future when asked to see people I know, I will casually answer general questions about their concerns (i.e. weight, cholesterol) in a public place rather than taking them under my clinical care. I will then not be privilege to additional medical or mental health information and possibly need to make treatment recommendations.

Practice Steps: Dual Relationships

1. Scan back through your experiences for the dual relationships in your practice. Pick out a few and remind yourself what the two relationships were. For example, your client was also your friend or your neighbor, or your student or doctor, etc.
2. Review how each part of the relationship began and notice if there were any points at which you had a clue that something didn't feel right. What was that feeling, a hesitation, dread, just an uncomfortable feeling?

3. Review how the relationship proceeded. Look at each separately. For example, if you counseled a friend, remember how the nutrition counseling progressed. Did the existence of the friendship affect the counseling? If so, how? Then remember the friendship. Did the fact that you were this person's nutrition counselor affect the friendship?
4. Is there anything you could have done to keep the boundaries clearer? Do you regret getting into that dual relationship?
5. What guidelines do you want to set for yourself going forward?
6. What can you learn from being on the other end of a dual relationship? Have you ever been the patient or client of a professional who was a friend? Were you honest and able to fully benefit from the consultation?

My Experiments With Dual Relationships

What I observe:

_____
_____
_____
_____
_____
_____
_____
_____

How I will experiment:

_____
_____
_____
_____
_____
_____
_____

Tip #14
Projection

If you hate a person, you hate something in him that is a part of yourself. What isn't part of ourselves doesn't disturb us.
Herman Hesse

When you judge another, you do not define them, you define yourself.
Wayne Dyer

Understanding the process of projection is useful for nutrition work. Projection is one of about 20 defenses. **Defenses are unconscious processes** that decrease anxiety caused by unacceptable thoughts or feelings. Unlike coping mechanisms, defenses tend to be rigid and compelled and do not respond to conscious choice. Everyone uses defenses. Each person has a few favorite defenses, and some are healthier than others.

Projection involves attributing to others unacceptable thoughts and/or feelings that one has but is not conscious of. Think of how **a movie projector** works. The projector is the person who has uncomfortable feelings or thoughts. The screen is the person onto whom the person projects the feelings or thoughts. The image (thoughts or feelings) is actually in the projector, but it appears to be on the screen. A person who is projecting is aware of the feelings or thoughts only in the other person, not in herself.

Clues that projection is happening:

* Someone states that she knows what someone else is feeling or thinking. How can she really know? She may be the one thinking or feeling this way and projecting onto the other.

* Your reaction to someone's statements about you is **puzzlement**. It doesn't make sense to you. It comes out of the blue. This is a clue that the person may be projecting onto you.

* There is an **unusual amount of energy** behind a statement someone makes about another. For example, your client goes on at length about someone else's behavior or characteristics.

Examples of projection:

* A client comes into a session and says, "You're going to hate me for this..." Unless you have shown strong negative judgments or hate toward her in previous sessions, this is projection. The client is projecting onto you her own strong negative judgments about her behavior.

* Someone who has **difficulty accepting her natural appetites** (whether for food or sex, or anything else) will project them in an exaggerated way onto others. For example, a client who is disgusted by seeing others eat may actually be conflicted about her own desire to eat.

* A large client complains of **strangers** who tell her what to eat or give her weight-loss suggestions. In this case, the strangers are projecting their own food and weight issues onto your client. Being projected upon can be very painful, especially if the implied judgment is one that the client has of herself.

* **Bigotry** of all kinds is driven by projection. The energy behind racism, for example, comes from the negative characteristics that the racist person has disowned and attributed to the "other."

What to do when you observe projection:

Not all projections need to be addressed. People hold on to their defenses rigidly, so trying to rip them away is generally ineffective or even cruel. Unless you are their therapist, it is **not your job** to help them take back projections. However, there are situations in which understanding the process can improve your work.

When someone is projecting onto your client and causing pain, you may have a role in **educating your client about the process of projection** and helping her with the skills to deflect it. You can explain the process and show her that it is all about what the other person is thinking/feeling about herself. Unfortunately, it tends to touch a nerve in the client that makes it feel true, so it is very difficult for her to take a larger perspective. I have sometimes found it helpful to speculate with the client what may be going on in the other person. Of course, we can never know for sure, but coming up with ideas may allow your client to deflect the projections more easily next time. For example, the teenagers who yelled out the window, "Fatty," may be feeling low esteem and need to put someone else down. The fellow gym member who offers unsolicited advice about sticking with exercise may be worried he will not be able to sustain his own program.

When a client is projecting onto you and it feels as if the work is affected, it is a good idea to address it. Gently ask supportive questions that cut through the projection. For example, when your client keeps assuming you are judging her negatively, you can ask her to state it clearly so you can respond with the truth. "You seem to imagine I am thinking some things about you. What exactly do you imagine I'm thinking?" If she is way off base, mirror her statements back to her. This may be enough to show her how irrational they are. If that's not enough, share a piece of what you are really thinking. I have often found myself saying, "Oh, that's what you imagined? That was the last thing on my mind. I was just thinking how persistent and committed you are to this process and that every time you have a setback we learn something new that is helpful to your progress."

Counter projection with simple, calm facts. You can practice this when acquaintances who know you are a dietitian project their food issues onto you. "You must think I'm a pig ordering a hamburger." Your response can be: "Actually, I was just trying to decide what I feel in the mood for. So, you're in the mood for a hamburger?" (For suggested language to counter projection with a client see page 110.)

When your **client seems to be projecting onto someone else** and she is stuck with it to the extent that you can't get anywhere in the session, acknowledge the strong feelings and redirect. For a therapist, this might be a perfect opportunity to direct the client toward her own feelings, but this isn't your role as the nutrition therapist. You could say, "Boy, you sure do feel strongly about that. Do you need to talk a bit more about that or would you like to use our time to work on your nutrition goals?" Acknowledge that it is hard to focus on (whatever it is you're trying to focus on: keeping records, figuring out how to exercise more, etc.) and gently redirect the client back.

Usually there is **a grain of reality** in the projection. It is important to acknowledge what is real first. In the above example, you could start by saying, "I see how that behavior would be annoying." Then you could move on to either redirect or to reality-check the projection.

Finally, **share what you observe** of the projection process with your client's therapist. The therapist may be able to work on it in therapy, and she may suggest some ideas for you. If you are in supervision, these are useful cases to bring up.

Case Study: A Client Who Projects Her Feelings Onto Others

Mary is a 40-year-old who has struggled with her weight and compulsive eating for many years. She told me several times that she holds back asking for what she needs in the way of food, especially with her family, believing that it would be "inconvenient" to them. I noticed that word, inconvenient, coming up over and over. At times, she also said it was inconvenient to stop to feed herself when she was alone.

One day we were reviewing a recent visit to her brother's house, and it came up again. I slowed her down and asked her to notice that word. She began to say again that she didn't want to inconvenience her brother and his wife by asking for a snack. I asked how she knew that this would inconvenience *them*. She couldn't point to any clues that this was true. I asked her if it seemed inconvenient *to her* to need food at that time. She said it certainly did, since there was no snack easily available.

Mary is slowly gaining practice at taking back this projection. I encourage her by mirroring back the feeling as it begins in her (It's a drag to stop to eat when I am busy). The next step is to invite her to let others determine what is and is not inconvenient to them. Here I may suggest she try some experiments that will keep her from projecting. (See Tip #3, Use of Experiments.)

Case Study: Helping a Client See Another's Projection

Judy is a 37-year-old who has had anorexia for most of her adult life. She has made significant progress and has not needed hospital admission since her mid-20s. She has insight about the role the eating disorder plays in the management of her anxiety and has learned how to manage the behaviors enough so that her health is not significantly affected. She is quite thin, though stable, and follows rigid rules for her eating.

She works in an office with a rich social life, and at least once a month, her department goes out to lunch together. She and I have worked hard on the best way to handle these events. She used to assume that everyone was looking at what she was eating (or not eating). She has finally taken that projection back and acknowledges that her extreme vigilance of her eating does not mean that others are paying such close attention, too. They are busy with their own thoughts and eating. She decides ahead what she will order that fits into her food plan, simply orders it, and then finds she can actually attend to the conversations at the table.

A few months ago, a new employee, Rona, began to make comments such as "Boy, I bet you can eat whatever you want." And, "Oh, you are being so good" (eating only salad for lunch). At first, Judy was just puzzled and didn't know what to say. We explored this, and she saw that the reason she felt so puzzled was that these comments did not relate at all to her experience. She certainly does not feel as if she can eat "whatever she wants." The eating disorder doesn't let her. Sticking to salad at lunch is not being "good," it's staying safe. Then Judy realized she felt angry at Rona. What right did she have to make these assumptions about Judy? I smiled and explained that, of course, she felt angry because Rona was projecting onto her. I briefly described projection.

I asked Judy if she had any clues as to what might cause Rona to focus on someone else's body and eating. Judy immediately could remember numerous times Rona had talked about her diets and her desire to lose weight. Judy is very intelligent and quickly put it together and said, "That's why she says these things! She wishes she could eat anything she wants and she thinks she is being bad eating what she eats. So, it's not about me, it's about her." I agreed. Now when Rona begins to talk about either her own eating or Judy's, Judy reminds herself that it's not about her, it's about Rona, and she finds an excuse to change the subject.

A few months later, Judy asked me why Rona always made these comments about her and rarely others in the department. I was about to make some suggestions when she asked if it might be because she was so thin. I told her this was likely. Someone will choose a person to project onto partly because of a characteristic that person has.

Guidelines for Responding to Projection

♦ Remind yourself of *who* you are, *what* you believe, what you *are* thinking. Stay grounded. (See page 34 for grounding techniques.)
♦ Mirror what you hear, adding "you imagine..." For example, "You imagine I think you are bad" or "You imagine that I am angry at you."
♦ Ask permission to correct it. "Would you be interested in hearing what I *was* thinking?"
♦ If the person seems willing and able to accept what is true for you, provide a few short statements of fact. Be honest and take care with how much you say. For example, "I was thinking how much progress you've made toward your goal of eating less often when you are not hungry." Or "I'm not angry at you. I *am* frustrated with how your eating disorder allows only small changes at a time. I believe you are frustrated for the same reason. Is that right?"
♦ Sometimes it is counterproductive to respond out loud at all. Often caring for oneself by grounding and getting out of the way of the projection is the best response.

Practice Steps: Projection

1. Spend a few days or weeks just searching for examples of projection. Review the clues in this Tip and see how many times you can spot the process happening.
2. Without actually doing or saying anything, begin to speculate about the possible factors that might have pushed the person to project. Assume that there was something going on that was uncomfortable for that person. You may speculate incorrectly, but at least you will be practicing looking at it as a process that begins in the person who is projecting.
3. Find a situation in which someone projects onto you frequently. Obvious examples might be the friend who assumes you are judging her because you are a nutrition professional or a specific client who often assumes you are thinking something you are not.
4. Prepare some handy statements of fact to try out the next time it happens. Try them out.
5. Review how your experiment went. Practice some more.

My Experiments With Projection

What I observe:

_____
_____
_____
_____
_____
_____

How I will experiment:

_____
_____
_____
_____
_____
_____
_____

Tip #15
Staying on Topic

We tell ourselves stories in order to live.
Joan Didion

*You've got to be careful if you don't
know where you're going,
because you might not get there.*
Yogi Berra

Mihn-Hai Tran, RD, of Dallas, asks how to keep consults focused on nutrition. "I get in situations where patients want to talk about their personal life, and it's a challenge to keep focused on the relevant topic." This is an issue for all of us at times.

A few thoughts about why this happens:

Some people **need to warm up** a bit before jumping right into the work. This can take the form of a monologue about their week or engaging you about a shared activity or interest. This can feel useless to you, but to clients, it may be essential to feel safe before addressing what they came in for.

Some people think **sequentially**. It's as if their brains store on reels of tape rather than a CD and they have to run through the whole tape with you before getting to the part where they need your help. This process can be frustrating for you, especially if your mind easily gets to the point. Those with **Attention Deficit Disorder** are easily distracted and find it difficult to maintain the thread of a conversation.

The topic may indeed be **more important** to your client at the moment than her food issues. For example, a client may come for a regularly scheduled visit just after an upsetting event. It may be impossible or even cruel to expect the client to go over food records two days after losing a close relative.

Finally, your client may be actively **avoiding the food issues** consciously or unconsciously. For example, a client comes in with deep ambiguity about making changes. The change of subject may be a smoke screen designed to protect her from uncomfortable feelings. This is the trickiest one to pick up on and to respond to. (You may want to review Tip #9 on Dealing With Resistance.)

Get clear yourself:

First, **notice your internal reaction**. Are you annoyed, angry, puzzled or frustrated? Any of these (and more) is normal. You are being thwarted in doing your job. Of course, you have a reaction. There are a few options here. You could expand your vision of what your job is, or you could set limits with your client. Or you could do some of each.

To expand the scope of your work, examine your willingness to be a sounding board for your client. There are times when the very best thing you can do for her is to **just be there**. Being a witness during tough times without demanding change is one of the most powerful things one human can do for another. Some of us have a larger capacity to do this than others. Know your limits. Once you know your capacity, the next step is to gain skill at communicating those limits to your client.

Setting limits is part of good nutrition counseling. Some sort of response is appropriate when your client spends much of the session on topics you do not believe further her nutrition goals. However, reacting and responding are two very different behaviors. Reacting out of your own feelings (frustration, for example) is not helpful to the client. Simply stating what is happening and asking your client to discuss it is an appropriate professional response.

Do you **hold back from redirecting** your client for fear of offending? Many of us were taught to be polite and not interrupt. It is part of our job to keep track of counseling goals (once they have been agreed upon), and sometimes that means interrupting and pointing out that the session is off target. That's not being impolite; it's being helpful.

What to do:

Dealing with this issue requires you to set aside the nutrition content and, for a moment, **attend to the process**. As dietitians, we are not used to doing this, but it doesn't mean we can't learn. It's appropriate for the process to become a brief topic of conversation between you and your client. When you've cleared the air, you can get back to the nutrition content.

Rather than pushing ahead with your agenda, go back to your client's. **Review what she came in with**. Direct the client's attention to the discrepancy between what she said she wanted from you and what you two are doing. There is a possibility you misinterpreted what your client really wanted, and this will bring out her true desire.

If it seems like a warming-up process, **mirror a bit** of what you are hearing and then ask if your client is ready to move on. "That's great that you had a fun weekend. Is it time to look at your food records?"

When an **unusual event** intrudes on the work, explicitly agree to limit your goals in this visit. "It sounds like working on your food goals today after this upsetting event is unrealistic. How about we just plan to spend the last 5 minutes to review where you are with your food and come up with one little goal this week? Right now I'd be glad to hear more if you need to talk. I'll let you know when we have 5 minutes left. Is that OK?"

Acknowledge any discomfort you notice in your client. Normalize her discomfort before moving on. "You seem to bring up something else when we begin to talk about your binge-and-purge episodes. I can understand how that would make you uncomfortable." This may be an opportunity to educate your client that getting better at tolerating discomfort is an essential step in recovery from an eating disorder. Your acceptance of the discomfort can provide a model for your client to adopt someday.

One strategy is to state what you see and then get curious. For example:

- "I hear that you are angry at your husband. I wonder if that relates to your evening eating."

- "I notice we often end up talking about your busy schedule. Is there a way I can help you adjust your schedule to allow you to reach your nutrition goals more easily?"
- "On the one hand I hear you saying you don't want to talk about these low blood-sugar episodes and on the other hand you came to me wanting to get your blood sugar under control. Are you curious about how these mixed feelings get in the way of your goals?"

If you often get off topic with the same client, suggest taking some time to **review how the sessions are going**. Ask for your client's assessment of what is working and what isn't. Then, add your observations:

- "I notice we keep going off the food issues. It's OK with me, but I do want to check in with you. Do you want me to direct us back or not?"
- "Might it be helpful to talk with a counselor about these issues? They sound important, and I'm not trained to help you resolve them."
- "Have you ever been evaluated for ADD?"
- "What do you value most about these sessions?"
- "Do you have others in your life to share these issues with?"

You may feel pressured by the limited number of visits allowed by insurance or by your employer. You don't have to take all the responsibility for making the best use of limited time. Talk about it with your client. If a client chooses to use the time in a way that seems like a waste to you, it's his choice. For example, "I'm aware that your insurance company will only cover three visits with me. How would you like to use this time?"

When all else fails, these excursions that clients take you on are perfect opportunities to **practice mirroring** (Tip #6). Mirroring invariably leads to some shift in the process.

If you're having trouble figuring out what is behind a particular client's getting off track, bring it up with a colleague or in supervision. You may need **an outside perspective** to see the process.

Case Study: Allowing a Client to Go Off Topic

Jennie Wade, MEd, RD, of Cincinnati, Ohio, shares this experience:

> As RDs, I think it's easy for us to believe that people come to us only for information on food, and that we need to "stick to the script." But I don't think that serves our clients.
>
> I recently had a woman come to me asking for advice on eating well to prepare for menopause and retain her energy levels as she grew older. In the third session, when she admitted to having some difficulty with the simple goals she had chosen, I asked her what might be in her way. By the end of the session, she was in tears talking about a lifelong friend who was draining all her energy. She seemed amazed at the emotions that bubbled up and realized that self-care would mean resolving a very stressful issue in her life.
>
> I'm so glad she felt comfortable talking with me. If I had been interested only in what she was eating, she would not have come to this important realization.

Sample Dialog: Using Changes of Subject to Help the Client

Molly: So, Sam, your food records show great progress with portions and stopping when you are satisfied.

Sam: Yes, I like paying attention to my appetite and also reminding myself that I will be eating again in a few hours. It really helps me push away from the table.

Molly: Great! Let's look at your exercise goals.

Sam: Well, right. You know the other day I actually left some food on my plate at a restaurant. I've never done that, but I thought of what you said about saving some for later and that worked.

Molly: You must be very pleased about that. How about your walking?

Sam: Last week, it rained a lot. As a matter of fact, did you realize that we had a total of 3 inches in four days! I have a rain gauge for my garden and I added up between Sunday and Wednesday. Isn't that amazing!

Molly: Yes, it is. Sam, I notice you change the subject when I bring up exercise. Shall we review whether that is still one of your goals?

Sam: Sure it is. I still get winded easily and I know it will help me lose weight. It's just that the food part is so much easier.

Molly: It's great that we've found ways to work on your portions that work so well for you. Of course, it's more fun to talk about success. I'm like that, too. It's a drag to take a look at the hard stuff. Sam, some of my clients avoid certain topics because they make them feel like a failure. Is that what's happening here?

Sam: Well, that's some of it. I know I am motivated best by seeing results. But maybe it's also because I don't like disappointing you. I hate to disappoint anyone.

This next section is also an example of one way to address projection, Tip #14.

Molly: Oh, so you imagine I am disappointed when you don't get your walks in? That's interesting.

Sam: Yes, you get so excited with me about the food stuff.

Molly: I'm not disappointed. Would you be interested in hearing my *real* reaction?

Sam: OK.

Molly: When you come in and tell me you didn't walk this week, first, I notice *your* disappointment. Then I find myself getting curious. Yes, I'm curious because I know it is important to you to be more active. So I am wondering what it is that gets in the way for you. I do want to help you figure it out, no matter how hard it is.

Sam: It is hard. I am so tired after work, and in the morning, it's still dark. Maybe I just can't do it during the week. I don't know why I can't do it on the weekends either, though.

Molly: Hmmm. Have you been expecting too much to start?

Sam: Yeah, maybe I've been figuring you want me to do it five days a week. I know it's still worth it to do it just a few. I'll see if I can walk this Saturday and Sunday. It's not supposed to rain.

Molly: And remember, I will not be disappointed no matter what. We'll get useful information from whatever happens.

Practice Steps: Staying on Topic

1. Think about your last few clients and pick out one with whom you have difficulty staying on the topic of nutrition. Look over the possible reasons for this in the Tip and make a guess which one (or ones) is most likely with this client.
2. Take a moment to notice your reaction to this client getting off track. Remember any reaction of yours is normal. Just notice it. Will it be useful and professional to share this response directly with the client? If not (for example, if you are angry) find someone to vent to and then go to step 3.
3. Pick a technique or two from the list in the Tip to try out with this client.
4. Observe the results and decide whether to continue this stance or try another one.

My Experiments With Staying on Topic

What I observe:

_____
_____
_____
_____
_____
_____
_____
_____
_____
_____
_____
_____
_____
_____

How I will experiment:

_____
_____
_____
_____
_____
_____
_____
_____
_____
_____
_____
_____
_____
_____

Tip #16
Handling Your Own Feelings
During a Session

*A professional is a person who can do his best
at a time when he doesn't particularly feel like it.*
Alistaire Cooke

Everything has something to teach you.
Wayne Dyer

It's normal to experience feelings toward clients. How we respond to these feelings is what distinguishes us as trained counselors. Some definitions will be helpful here:

Transference is the experience of feelings, drives, attitudes and defenses toward a person in the present that do not fit that person but are a repetition of reactions originating in the past, unconsciously displaced onto figures in the present. Therapists use this term to refer to a client's experience. Example: A college-age client begins to resist all of the nutritionist's ideas and behaves rebelliously, just as she did with her parents when she was a teen.

Countertransference refers to your reactions to the client. There are two kinds of countertransference. The first involves your feelings, drives, attitudes and defenses that you transfer onto the client from other parts of your life. If not contained, these can interfere with the counseling and need to be addressed in supervision. Sometimes this is called **subjective** countertransference. It clouds your view of the client and does not allow you to truly see her as she is.

114

The other kind of countertransference refers to reality-based reactions to the client's behavior. These may be a source of insight into the client. They can be called **objective** countertransference. Both kinds of countertransference can be positive or negative.

Examples of subjective countertransference:

You are on a limited budget and feel **jealous** of a client who is wealthy. You may have **judgments** about how she spends her money.

You may be feeling **unsuccessful** and need the next client to make progress to confirm your competence.

You find yourself thinking about **your own issues** with food, diet and your body as your client talks about hers. This can interfere with your ability to fully understand and accept your client.

Your client **reminds you of someone** about whom you have strong feelings. This can be anything from anger or fear to concern or sexual attraction.   If you begin to behave as if your client is that other person, it will confuse your client and harm the work.

If you **identify with your client,** it is easy to transfer the feelings and desires you had at her stage of life onto her. This may help you understand her. You also run the risk of missing some important differences.

You may make **assumptions** based on your experience with previous clients or your beliefs about how the counseling process is supposed to go. This can hold a client back from following her path to change.

It is not unusual to feel **angry** at a client.   Sounding or acting angry is not helpful to the client.

Having warm, **caring feelings** toward clients can be one of the joys of any kind of counseling. You are motivated to do your best when you care about clients, their lives and their outcomes. It's wonderful to feel useful and appreciated. These positive feelings are a problem only if your need to be useful begins to interfere with what the clients need. For example, when a favorite client leaves treatment, it is normal to experience loss. It may be tempting to persuade the client to stay. Working to help clients determine what's best for them in spite of how it will affect you is the professional approach.

Examples of objective countertransference:

Feelings of **resentment** could be a clue that the client is expecting too much and/or you are working too hard.

When you feel **bored** in a session, it could mean the client is not connecting with you. She probably is skirting issues and not connecting with much of importance to herself, either.

Uncomfortable feelings you experience while disclosing something about yourself could be a clue that this is not a safe or wise move for you and/or your client. (See Tip #1, Self-Disclosure.)

Feeling confused, overwhelmed or helpless could mean that the client is feeling that way, too.

If you are in a **dual relationship** with your client, your feelings of discomfort are accurate clues that more discussion is needed or that a portion of the relationship needs to end. (See Tip #13, Dual Relationships.)

When you feel yourself **pushing or arguing** with your client, this is a reliable indicator of resistance. (See Tip #9, Dealing With Resistance.)

You may experience anxiety or fear after hearing a client describe **a traumatic experience.** In this case, you are experiencing secondary trauma, a normal reaction to witnessing someone else's trauma. If the client's story causes you to remember trauma in your past, this would be an example of subjective countertransference mixed in.

What to do when you become aware of a feeling:

First, acknowledge it to yourself. All feelings are acceptable. What you do with the feeling is what matters. The sooner you can put a word or phrase on the feeling, the more you are able to respond in a professional manner. **Reacting** in the moment without thought is generally not productive. **Responding** after considering how your words and/or behavior will affect the client is professional. **Reacting** is knee-jerk and usually out of fear, hurt or anger; **responding** involves choice. A useful question to ask yourself is if what you plan to say or do is for the client's benefit or yours. If you cannot figure out whether your words are going to be useful, it's best to contain them.

Later, **in a quiet moment,** take yourself back to that difficult moment in the session. When the client is not there, you may be able to put a word on the feeling and learn from it. If it's "your stuff" popping up, make a note to see if it repeats. If the same feelings keep coming up in sessions or with a certain client and it's getting in the way for you, consider bringing it up with a supervisor or in your own therapy.

For example, consider feelings that are triggered in an **empathetic response** to your client. She may be talking about the death of her mother just before her bulimia started and you feel a heavy feeling in your chest and maybe some tears in your eyes. You are remembering your losses. Briefly and silently, acknowledge your own feelings and remind yourself that this session is about her, not you, then acknowledge her feelings. (See Tip #6, Mirroring.) If you must say something about your response because it is obvious (for example, you are visibly crying), keep your comment short and client-focused. For example, "As you see, I can identify with that." Remember that your empathetic response is normal and wonderfully human. However, making the session about you and your feelings is not professional.

It may be best to **avoid certain types of cases.** If you discover that you are easily triggered by certain clients and you have difficulty staying in your professional role, consider screening such clients out of your practice. Keep a list of colleagues for referrals. Acknowledging your limits is one of the best things you can do for your clients. Some therapists will not see sexual-abuse survivors, for example, because they find it too difficult to contain their responses.

Examples of how to use objective countertransference:

Resentment is one of the most useful feelings humans experience. It is the feeling you have when a "no" should have been said or a request should have been made. Consider the client who asks you to schedule her after your regular office hours. If you agree and then feel resentment, this means a necessary boundary was stepped over. Letting this happen again and again with one client will cause resentment to build up and the work will be compromised. Some clients push you again and again. They need you to set careful limits. When you do set the necessary limits, it pays off for you and for them. Of course, there are times when you agree to go out of your way for clients and don't feel resentment. This indicates that your boundaries were not breached.

When you wonder whether your client is **feeling confused, overwhelmed or helpless** because you are, go through a few quick steps in your head. First, take a deep breath and figuratively step back into a place of professional competence. Remind yourself that you do not always feel so helpless. Recall a time you felt self-assured. Next, consider asking your client how she feels right now. You could add that you suspect she might be feeling confused/overwhelmed/helpless. If she confirms your guess, validate her experience for a moment and then move on to provide the clarity, direction or hope that she may lack right now. Especially with an eating-disorder client, your role may include holding hope when she can't.

Some situations include both types of countertransference. For example, if a client is frustrated with a lack of progress toward his goals and **accuses you of not being a good dietitian**, it would be quite normal for you to feel inadequate and defensive. However, the session isn't about you; it's about the client and his goals. The strength of your feeling of incompetence may reflect the strength of his feelings of incompetence or frustration. The most professional way to respond is to tuck away your feelings (noting how strong they are) and keep the conversation on his frustration and what to do next. This may be especially hard if you are carrying leftover feelings of inadequacy from your family or from other parts of your career. (See Tip #5, How to Respond to Your Client's Strong Feelings, for other ideas.)

Case Study: Subjective Countertransference

Donna Foster, RD, of Lexington, Ky., called to consult with me about a case. She had been seeing Allan weekly for six months. He was a 17-year-old with Type 1 diabetes. One year ago, he decided to address being a little overweight. He began restricting and kept losing weight to well below ideal. He was stuck in a pattern of restricting and occasionally binging. He tested his blood sugar regularly and was in only moderate control. He was in therapy and expressed a desire to get his life back and go back to school. He had also shared that he is gay and that no one knows except his mother, his therapist and the dietitian. Donna's concern was that she found herself angry at him for continuing to not eat enough and not care for his diabetes. She knew that acting angry would be unprofessional and would not be useful to the client.   She felt angry often in Allan's sessions and worried that her feelings would slip out.

I congratulated her for noticing her anger and being willing to look at it.   She knew that she had other clients who were as frustrating, but she didn't get this angry with them.   She wondered why she got so angry at Allan.

We talked about anger for a few minutes.   I reminded her that anger is what we feel when things are not going the way we want them to.   The more we care about something, the angrier we get if it doesn't happen.   I could hear the anger in her voice. She agreed that she had more energy when she thought of him than most of her clients.   I asked her to notice the energy and see if she could sense where it came from in her.   She quickly realized that she cared deeply about Allan.   He was engaging, bright and interesting.   She was fearful he would not recover and would not "get his life back."   She admitted being sad about this possibility. I reminded her that she can't control what Allan does.   She admitted not liking that lack of control but readily acknowledged it.   As is often the case, this dietitian's anger was masking several layers of feeling.   In her case, it was caring about the client, sadness that he might not live out his dreams, and helplessness at what she could not change.

We ended the call after she reviewed the ways to care for herself and let go of what she can't control.

Here's another example of subjective countertransference worked through well. Stephanie Brooks, MS, RD, of Campbell, Calif., sent this:

I had a 12-year-old girl with anorexia as a client. In our first session, I had a hard time focusing and keeping on track with the intake.   I kept having this feeling that I'd rather be going to Starbucks or a movie with her than sitting in my office doing this. At first, I just dismissed it as my needing a break.

During our next session, similar thoughts came into my mind. I'd rather be doing something else with this girl. I wanted to talk about her interests regarding school, friends, hobbies. ... In fact, we did spend a longer than usual time discussing those things. At the end of the session, when she was leaving, I found myself wanting to give her a big hug. ...I didn't though.

I spoke to the client's therapist, with whom I have a long working relationship, and explained what I was thinking and feeling. I asked if she was feeling the same way, thinking maybe it was something about this client. The therapist responded that she hadn't had these thoughts. Later that night, I was talking with my husband about some plans we had with his family and it struck me that this client reminded me of my 13-year-old niece. I can't believe I didn't figure this out earlier. They look, speak and smile similarly. Their sense of humor and personalities are close as well.

I called the client's therapist and explained why I was feeling the way I was. We discussed if it would be good for me to stay on the case. The client did feel comfortable with me and was making good progress. If I referred her to a colleague, would she be able to connect with another nutrition therapist and do as well? We decided that since I hadn't acted out any of my thoughts or feelings and that I now knew where they were coming from, it would be OK to stay on the case. I would need to be more aware of my thoughts.

I ended up working with this client for about two years. As our time together progressed, I no longer saw her as my niece, but as my client. It was challenging in the beginning to stay focused and on task. I also came to realize that when these thoughts entered my mind, it was time to visit my niece.

Case Study: Objective Countertransference

In these two cases, the dietitian's feelings provided useful information that was then used in the treatment process.

One day in my supervision group, a dietitian came in saying she needed help with a family she was working with. She specializes in pediatrics, and this family had been referred by a pediatrician because the 8-year-old son was gaining weight rapidly. She was extremely frustrated with the parents and vented for a few minutes about how many times they had called at the last minute to reschedule an appointment, or had come late or brought the younger children even after all agreed that wasn't productive. We could have looked into the details of the boy's eating habits and food choices, but I urged her to stay with her experience with the family so we could learn from it. She was clearly having strong feelings, so this was an example of countertransference. To help us see how much was objective, I checked with the others in the group. Every one of us (including myself) agreed that we would react similarly to such a family. This was a good clue that the dietitian's feelings were more about the family than about herself or her past. So, I proceeded to further explore her feelings for useful insights into the case and how best to proceed.

We worked to unpack all of the dietitian's frustrations. What emerged was her sense that the family was not allowing her to do her job. I pointed out that indeed they were doing everything possible to stifle her. Of course, any professional would be annoyed. Looking at it from the family's perspective, this behavior pattern can be seen as resistance to change. They continued to schedule sessions, indicating some desire to work on the issue. Then their resistance came forward again. This pattern shows ambivalence. We were also able to see the pattern of cancellations as reflecting the chaos in this family that was likely affecting the children. She decided that if the parents managed to come to another session, she would point out the ambivalence she was seeing and offer a referral to a family therapist who could help them cope with their busy lives.

In this case, careful attention to my emotions helped me and this client work more effectively together.

A few years ago, I got a call from, Karl, a 30-year-old man for weight control. The initial scheduling phone call took 30 minutes, much longer than usual. By our fourth session, I was feeling angry and resentful. He often brought up important issues just as our time was up and twice called me between sessions to ask questions that I thought could wait until our appointment time.

Because of my emotional reaction to Karl, I suspected he had a personality disorder. I had a signed release to talk with his therapist of several years. She said that her working diagnosis was Generalized Anxiety Disorder and Borderline Personality Disorder. She confirmed my plan to maintain firm boundaries with this client. I reminded myself to set and maintain clear limits on session length, fee payment, and the number of calls between sessions. For a while, I needed to be deliberate and very clear about these limits. After a month or so, he needed fewer reminders. My resentment went down, and he seemed to be more comfortable.

Practice Steps: Handling Your Own Feelings

1. Observe all you can about your feelings toward clients. First, just note them. Give them a word or phrase and jot them down.
2. See if you can distinguish your feelings transferred from other parts of your life from the ones that are a normal, expected response to the client's behavior.
3. If you can pinpoint feelings that are transferred from elsewhere, simply being aware of this may be enough. If your feelings continue to get in the way of staying professional with your client, bring it up with a supervisor or therapist.
4. If you believe your feelings are normal given this client, find ways to glean useful information from your reactions. You may need to ask a supervisor to help you.
5. Puzzled by some of your reactions to clients? Bring them up with a colleague or in supervision. Talking about it out loud can help you sort it out. Emotional reactions to clients are some of the hardest issues to bring up in supervision. They are also the most useful!

My Experiments With Using My Feelings

What I observe:

_____
_____
_____
_____
_____

How I will experiment:

_____
_____
_____
_____
_____

Tip #17
Asking "How" and "What"
Instead of "Why"

The aspects of things that are most important to us are hidden because of their simplicity and familiarity.
Ludwig Wittgenstein

It is better to know some of the questions than all of the answers.
James Thurber

You may find yourself asking, "Why":

- "Why does this client keep overeating?"
- "Why can't he understand that blood sugar testing is important?"
- "Why can't my anorexic client just start eating more?"
- "Why do so few of my clients come for follow-up visits?"
- "Why does she binge and purge?"
- "Why can't I attract more clients?"
- "Why do I keep making the same mistake with a certain type of client?"

You may be genuinely curious about the cause, but more likely, you just want the situation to change. If that's the case, change the wording of your questions to begin with "how" or "what." You may be surprised with the results.

Language Shift Ideas

INSTEAD OF:	EXPERIMENT WITH:
Why did you binge?	*What* was happening just before the binge? *How* did you feel a few minutes before you went into the kitchen? *How* do these overeating episodes begin? *What* happens next? *What* is going through your mind at the times you are able to eat a normal dinner?
Why won't you keep your food records anymore?	*What* is it like for you when you bring records in to me? *What* gets in the way of writing down your foods? *How* do you feel when you look at what you have eaten for a day?
Why can't you ask your friend to stop commenting on your weight?	*What* is your reaction when she says that? *How* does it affect your eating? *What* do you *feel* like saying to her? *How* would you prefer she relate to you?
Why don't you bring your lunch to work?	*What* do you dislike about packing a lunch? *How* would it be to get to lunchtime and find a packed lunch ready for you? *What* foods do you most want for lunch at work? If you did pack a lunch, *how* would you do it? *What* would you include?
Why won't you eat any fat?	*What* do you fear eating fat will do? *How* did you feel when you had to eat it in the hospital? *What* happened? Do you know *what* the fat in your food does for you?
Why don't you test your blood sugar every day the way the doctor wants you to?	*What* matters to you most about your diabetes? *How* do you see blood sugar results helping you? What gets in the way of testing? *How* is it so easy for you to brush your teeth every day? *What* stands in the way of relating to blood sugar testing that way?
Why is my practice so slow?	*How* did the clients whom I like working with find me? *How* do I interact with the clients who come back?

These questions work better because:

- "Why" often implies judgment. Judgment and condemnation do not contribute to change; they actually make change less likely. "How" **assumes acceptance** of what is. It encourages acceptance and observation of what is happening, a necessary first step toward doing something different.

- You **can always get answers** to "how" or "what" questions. At times, the subconscious mind will not let out the reason why for something. The reasons may be too complicated or too scary. Staying with the process questions helps you avoid resistance. You rarely run into defense mechanisms when you ask "how" or "what."

- That's **where all the useful answers are**. Knowing *why* a behavior is happening rarely leads to positive change. Knowing in detail *what* happens and precisely *how* it happens gets at the *process* that results in the behavior under question. By pursuing the details of a process (how and what), you can see a path to new behaviors.

- This type of questioning leads you and your client to **look at the issue or problem from many angles**. You never know what will pop up. Useful information or perspectives will emerge that allow you to make progress toward your goals.

- These questions encourage a **state of open curiosity**. The longer you can stay curious about the process and not assume you know everything about it, the more you will help your client.

Practice Steps: "Why?" vs. "How?" and "What?"

1. Spend a week looking for the times you start a thought or a sentence with "Why?"
2. When you are ready, begin to catch yourself before the word comes out. Take a breath and find a way to ask the same thing in a series of "how" and "what" questions.
3. Notice what happens.

My Experiments With Why?, How? and What?

What I observe:

_____
_____
_____
_____
_____
_____
_____
_____
_____
_____
_____

How I will experiment:

_____
_____
_____
_____
_____
_____
_____
_____
_____
_____
_____
_____
_____

Tip #18
How To Handle Personal Questions

Whatever you expect,
it will be different.
The Buddha

It is better to know some of the questions
than all of the answers.
James Thurber

All of us have been asked personal questions in the course of nutrition counseling. Here are a few examples from my practice:

- Have you ever been heavy?
- Do you have diabetes, too?
- Who are you voting for in the election this fall?
- Are you married?
- Do you have children?
- How can you stand listening to people's problems all day?
- Are you a Christian?
- How do you eat?
- Where do you and your husband like to go out to eat?

There is one principle to follow in responding:

The question is **not about you**; it's about your client.

Here are the steps I take:

First, I quickly check in with myself to see whether I am willing to disclose this information. Some areas are just too personal or my answer will not be in the client's best interest. Deciding whether to share personal information with clients is your choice. There is no reason you should feel you have to answer just because you are asked. Many professionals never answer personal questions. If you feel comfortable answering, make sure the way you answer furthers the work you are there to do.

If I am willing to let the client know that, for example, I have a son, I will say, "I'd be glad to answer that, but first I'm **curious where that question comes from.**" Often the response is something like, "I want to know if you can understand how hard it is to get picky children to eat well." Once I find out what matters to the client, I respond to that first and then briefly answer her question. For example, "Oh, I do know that this is really hard. My son is 20 now, and I remember that stage very well. It's really frustrating. I also remember worrying I wasn't being a good parent. Is that how you are feeling, or is it something else?" Notice in this example I continue trying to understand what is bothering the client. I tell her about my experience as a parent, but only to clarify her concern. Then I can reassure or give specific guidance that speaks to her present need.

If **I do not share the client's experience** and I am willing to disclose this, I follow the same format. For example, "I hear that keeping track of your diet to control your blood sugar is really hard and so many people in your life just don't understand. That must be maddening. I don't have diabetes, but I can relate to that experience of not being understood about something so important."

Questions about the **dietitian's weight or eating-disorder history** are tricky. For some dietitians, the model used in the above examples may work. This would mean a very brief answer about your experience within the context of what the client needs at the moment. For example, "Yes, I have struggled with my weight at times, and I remember well this stage you are in. It is hard to keep in mind the big picture." Or, if you are not willing to disclose your experience, redirect the client by asking what she imagines your answer would do for her. There may be a way to provide what she needs without disclosure.

As health professionals, most of us have struggled to practice what we preach. When we are successful, it is tempting to **act as models for our clients.** Your story may be a powerful educational tool and support to some clients. For others, it could discourage them or not allow them to find their unique path of change. There is a handy way to evaluate if you are using your experience appropriately: notice whether you tell your story to most of your clients and in the same way each time. If so, you are most likely off base with some of them. Consider withholding your story until you have heard more about their struggle.

If you have a **story that will truly help your client**, first find out if the advice is wanted (see Tip #4, Asking Your Client for Ideas on page 17), then put it in general terms rather than bringing "I" into the conversation. For example, you want to tell your client about an idea that works well for you. Instead of saying, "I put my workout clothes by my bed so it will be easy in the morning," ask whether she is ready for suggestions, then say, "You may want to consider putting out..." Then you can ask for a response to this idea, and the focus remains on the client.

When it comes to **religion and politics**, I choose to dodge those questions completely. If my client and I have very different views, my response could turn her off and I would lose the rapport that is so valuable. The purpose of this relationship has nothing to do with politics or religion, so I choose to avoid this distraction. It is your choice. Just be aware of the pitfalls.

Sometimes a **question has an assumption embedded** in it. For example, if a client asks me where my husband and I like to eat out, the client is assuming that I have a husband and that we like to eat out. One of these is not true in my case, but there is no reason to correct the client. It's more important to figure out where the question comes from and address that. For example, "I have an answer for you on that, but first it would help me to understand what it is you are looking for here." He could be looking for healthy places to eat or trying to gain my approval for how often he eats out, or something else I don't have a clue about until I hear it from him.

A basic format to follow:

- Figure out what you are willing to disclose.
- Bring out where the question comes from and what's behind it.
- Respond to what matters to the client.
- Very briefly self-disclose (if you are willing to).
- Word your answer so that it serves the client's needs.
- Redirect the topic back to the client.

When clients ask personal questions, the issues are often the same ones that arise when   you volunteer information about yourself during counseling. (See Tip #1, Self-Disclosure, for more ideas.)

A Conversation on Handling Personal Questions

One day on a group phone supervision call this topic came up. Here's an edited version of our discussion:

> **Marcy Fiacco, MS, RD:** I was working with a weight-control client the other day. She and I are about the same age, so I can identify with her. One day, during a follow-up session, she asked me how much I weigh. I thought for a second, "am I going to answer this? She probably thinks she should know mine since I know hers." I just said, "Well, you know, I would say I'm a dress size and pant size above where I'd like to be," and that's the way I left it. Afterward, I wondered from your therapist perspective, Molly, what she was trying to do?
>
> **Molly:** That's a really interesting situation, isn't it? And it's hard to know to what extent you inadvertently invited her to do that.
>
> **Marcy:** I guess I did.
>
> **Molly:** Mentioning your stuff about body and weight certainly builds rapport in a friend-to-friend relationship. Here it told her that it was OK to ask about your weight.
>
> **Marcy:** What would you do?
>
> **Molly:** I would first ask, "What do you hope my answer will do for you?" Marcy, do you have any idea what she would have said?
>
> **Marcy:** I'm not sure. We are similar height and age, and maybe she wanted to
> compare her level of success with weight control with mine. I really don't know what she wanted from me.
>
> **Molly:** I believe it's valid to ask a client: "What would you like from that? Where is that question coming from?" I may be willing or not to talk about my weight. That's a whole different issue that

is mostly mine. What's more important is that by saying a number, I don't think I'm answering the person's question. Remember that the question is not about you – your body, your number on the scale today – and it isn't, frankly, about your being a little uncomfortable with your size and wanting to be a size smaller. It's about her – because it's her session – it's about her struggle with size and weight and figuring out if she's an OK person and whatever else is involved there for her. When somebody throws out a blunt question like that, it doesn't get at the real issue.

Elyssa Hurlbut, MS, RD: Molly, when Marcy asked you what you would do, my first inclination was to say that I would ask the client, "Why do you want to know that?" Or, "Why are you asking?" Then I realized that this would cause her to be defensive.

Molly: Because of that word "why"?

Elyssa: Yes, so that clearly was not the right question to ask.

Molly: It's the right *type* of question because it gets at what's behind her question. Let me slow down here and tell you what I think when someone asks me a personal question. There's something important for the client, or she would not have asked me about my body. I also know that the question is not about *my* body, Molly's body; it's about something very important to her and I can't answer the question yet because I don't know what the real question is. So I need to ask more questions to find out what this person really wants from me. I could hand her my weight – the number – and it would likely fall flat. Once the client asks something I can answer, I do.

Marcy: It was interesting because I've been in the field a million years it seems like, but I've never had anybody throw that particular question at me. I thought it was unusual, because actually, for my age, I think I look pretty good. So it's not something I would generally hear. I could see that she was comparing because of our similar ages and height and stuff.

Molly: The fact that you are rarely asked that question is another clue that it is all about the client. You don't know what the real issue is until you unpack it. For example, it might be, "I'm always comparing myself to other people and I want to know if I look as good as them or better than them." You could choose to use your own body as an example if you want to. But it might work better to shift it to talking about the client's friends, sisters, cousins, etc. The problem is that if you do answer a specific question, the client then knows "my dietitian is 5'6" and weighs 140 pounds." That's so concrete and so tied up with "my dietitian, the expert." She can't help but set you up as a model, and does that help her?

Marcy: I was sitting there thinking if she was trying to decide that I'm not going to be able to help her because my weight is OK. Do you have any good lines for the client who looks at you and says, "Well, you never had a weight problem, so why should I listen to you?"

Molly: And sometimes they don't even allow you to answer. A client might say, "Oh you don't have to worry about weight" or "You don't have to watch what you eat."

Marcy: They're telling you they're not open to anything you say. It seems like they want to discredit you at the beginning. I'm talking about situations where you have just met this person, maybe someone who's in an orientation about a weight-control program. The very first thing they say is, "I don't think you're going to be able to help me lose weight because you obviously have never had a weight problem."

Molly: Marcy, would you be interested to hear my response to that? I've certainly gotten that kind of thing. My response would be to mirror. I would pick a few words or phrases and I would mirror them back. For instance, "Oh, it sounds to me like it's really important if you join this program that you are understood. You would want me and the other people in the group to know how hard this is. Is that right?" That's an example.

Marcy: So it's never about you.

Molly: I'm going on the assumption it isn't about me. Particularly if someone is saying, "You don't understand." There's no way I'm going to win an argument about whether I understand. Why get into an argument about it? It doesn't get anywhere. Instead, I put it back on the client and simply acknowledge how much they want to be understood. I can understand that. If it's someone I already know a little bit, I'll go the next step of asking, "So far as we work together, does it sound like I get at least some of what you're going through?" If I'm meeting them new, there is no experience to draw on, but I might say, "It's really important to me, too, that if you're in this group, you feel that people around you get it and that I get at least part of what's going on for you. So I want to ask you a favor. If at any point I say something that sounds like I don't get it, will you tell me?" Marcy, I'm serious when I say that because I know I'm not totally attuned all the time and I want to be called on it. Does that feel helpful?

Marcy: I think that really empowers them. I like that. I found myself defensive and saying, "Well, I've had three kids and I've gained 35 pounds each time, and I've had to work every bit of those 35 pounds off after each pregnancy."

Molly: Exactly. All that stuff is absolutely true and it is part of *your* story, and what good does it do your client?

Judith Mabel, RD, PhD: The struggles I've been through don't do them any good 'cause they're not their struggles. I lost weight a few years ago and my mood was affected. I put it back on again. I have some kind of a brain hormonal imbalance that wouldn't let me lose the weight. It's not their business. It's not their problem.

Molly: Exactly! And we each have our wonderfully complex, true, real struggles and stories. Now, Judy, to take that specific example, there may be an opportunity someday for you to make use of your experience with a client. You may be able to share that sometimes a person loses enough weight or rapidly enough that their mood goes down and their body doesn't want them to be at that weight. So you might be able to share that with someone, but you're not telling your story.

Let's get back to when clients assume that either we won't understand or that we're perfect and it's easy for us. It can be helpful to first bring out the clients' assumptions and find out exactly what they're assuming.

Elyssa: How do you do that in a way that's not invasive and that comes across as natural?

Molly: Here's an example: "Hold on a minute. You just said that I don't need to watch what I eat. Let's talk about that. It sounds important to you and it would help me to understand more about what you are assuming about my eating. I think I hear that you figure I just go about my day and eat whatever I want and don't think about it at all. Is that what you're saying?" I mirror back what I hear the client saying. The client is saying something about herself or her doubts or what it is she fears she won't get from you. It may feel scary to ask the client to clearly give you her doubts. I find once I get what the doubts and concerns are, it's easy to answer. If instead I try to answer the big challenge that "you can't help me," I get lost and defensive. If they say, "I'm really doubtful that you can help me because I've been to three other dietitians before and they haven't helped," that clearly isn't about you.

Elyssa: I don't know if this is getting defensive, but I might also say something about the positives of working with somebody like a dietitian because we have training. Because we're successful with many people and because we see the ups and downs a person goes through during this process, or is that being too defensive?

Molly: It may come across as defensive because it is about *your* expertise and experience, and I don't think it's possible to win that argument. How do you know how to answer if you can help the client unless you have a clear idea of what her doubts are? It's helpful to have a phrase to say first so you can collect your thoughts. When it's a personal question, the phrase that I automatically spit out is, "Oh, so what you're asking is..." And then if I'm willing, I'll say, "That's something I'm willing to answer." But I don't answer it yet. Those few sentences help me collect my thoughts about what clarifying questions I need to ask.

It's a clue I'm getting defensive when I feel like saying, "Wait a minute, just because I'm a dietitian doesn't mean I..." That's when I need to take a deep breath and think, OK, this energy is coming from the client, there's some big deal for them here and they're projecting onto me.

Elyssa: It's interesting because we've come up with different motivations for why a client would ask us a question.

Molly: Oh, they're all over the map.

Elyssa: What we haven't said was that they just want to bond better. They want more camaraderie with us. More rapport, such as "We're really alike. That's why I can work with you, because we have similar situations. You have children and you know how difficult it is to x, y and z..."

Molly: And you may be absolutely right. When they ask, "How do you handle coming home from a long day of work and cooking dinner?" That isn't about you and your house and your children and your food. It's about how they handle it and how tough it is. You're absolutely right – sometimes it's just wanting validation. I believe that in a professional relationship there are better ways to validate a client's experience than self- disclosure.

That gets us back to Marcy's case. You noticed that it was right after you had been rapport-building that the client asked a personal question. Marcy, you might want to experiment here. When you feel like saying friendly, validating things about your size or your age, see if it's possible to validate the client's experience without saying anything about yourself. It is not uncommon after self-disclosure to get in the kind of trap you did.

Judy: Well, you could say something like, "Yeah, it truly is a juggling act when people have a job and children" without saying, "I'm having the same trouble in this particular area."

Molly: Yes, mirroring it back in your own words. Slightly changing the words, "And wow, and after a tough day, it is hard, isn't it?" or "Boy, I'll bet your kids are giving you a hard time. " That way you do respond, but keep it their story.

Marcy: Thank you, I really appreciate that because that was the first time I'd ever gotten that one.

Judy: This brings up something that I deal with. I never was overweight until after my second child was born, and now weight loss is very, very difficult for me. I'm wondering if there's anything I should do or just keep seeing the clients who choose to see me. If they want this perfect figure, then they'll obviously take one visit and go elsewhere. I don't see many weight-loss clients. I'd like to see more because there's more out there.

Marcy: I think that you lose either way. In my experience, I find that if you're overweight, they'll say that you don't know what you're doing because you're overweight. But if you're thin, they'll say you'll never understand because you obviously don't have a weight problem.

Molly: I don't have any hard and fast rule about bringing it up yourself if the client doesn't. I think a lot of clinicians don't bring it up. If it does come up, be willing to find out what it means for the client. It could be extremely interesting.

Judy: It's never come up. Nobody has ever said, "you're a little more than I expected."

Molly: Have you ever had a situation, Judy, where you suspected they were thinking something like that because of something they said?

Judy: There probably were a couple of times my ears perked up, but I don't remember.

Molly: If you're ever suspecting it, you can at least open a door to indicate it would be OK if the client said something about the effect of your particular body on the work with you. You always keep it in terms of it being about the work and the effect of your particular body on their process. Their process is what matters.

Judy: I'm hoping to do a weight-loss group. I'm finding names and putting a group together, and my assumption is it will come up as we meet and get to know each other week after week.

Molly: And people will have assumptions. Let's say you are three weeks in and there are six people in the group. A few will have come to the conclusion that you're someone who used to be a lot heavier and because of all these wonderful techniques you're teaching them you have lost weight. And there will be other clients who are thinking, I'm not sure any of these are good ideas because look at her. Their thoughts have more to do with their hope and their self-efficacy than with you.

Nancy D. Smith, MS, RD, CDE: Is there ever a time when it's appropriate for a dietitian to self-disclose something about themselves?

Molly: Yes. If the self-disclosure or answering the personal question is indeed going to be in the service of the client. I am incapable of knowing whether it's going to be in service of the client until I've asked some follow-up questions. The other caveat is that whatever you disclose, do so as a sound bite, so you can keep an eye on the client and notice her response and encourage her to tell you her response. If you go on and on about your story, the whole session becomes about you, and that isn't the point. It's the client's session.

Case Study: A Rare Example of Answering a Personal Question

Several years ago, I worked with a client recovering from bulimia for over a year. She asked me several times about my weight or made comments on my body. In each case, I didn't answer her question, I unpacked it instead and useful information emerged. She was obsessed with her weight, which, according to weight-for-height charts, was on the higher end of normal for her height.

After many months, I realized that it might be helpful for her to have a reality check and that using my body might work. Over several sessions, I asked her what she sees when she looks at my body. Of course, I had to be comfortable with that and not take any of it personally. I had to step back and treat my body sitting in that room as if it were a photograph. It's not me, Molly, it's a prop that we're using in the service of the client. By going slowly, we were able to do that.

It was helpful for her partly because she has a body similar to mine. I am fairly large-boned and muscular. That body type comes from my family. My weight for height on the charts looks high just like hers, even though my body composition is 17% body fat. (I didn't share that number with my client because I feared encouraging competition.) She had already told me she saw me as lean, the way she wanted to be. I knew our body types were similar and guessed that she would find it useful to know there are other bodies like hers. By taking it slowly we accomplished that. It wasn't about my body. It was in the service of her figuring out her body.

If this client had shown characteristics of Borderline Personality Disorder or other indications that she had difficulty distinguishing between herself and others, I would not have tried this.

Practice Steps: Personal Questions

1. Find some wording that feels comfortable for your initial response to personal questions.
2. Commit the words to memory.
3. Think about the types of questions you have been asked and the ones you most fear. Are you willing to answer them if you decide it is in the service of the client? My suggestion is to begin with a default approach of planning to not disclose unless there is a compelling reason to.
4. Wait until a client asks you a personal question.
5. Begin with your chosen words (even if they don't quite fit). As you catch your breath, begin to unpack the client's question.
6. Stay curious about what is there for the client.
7. Debrief the experience afterward with a colleague or supervisor.

My Experiments With Personal Questions

What I observe:

_____
_____
_____
_____
_____

How I will experiment:

_____
_____
_____
_____
_____

Tip #19
How a Mindfulness Practice Aids Our Work

*In the attitude of silence the soul finds
the path in a clearer light, and what is elusive
and deceptive resolves itself into crystal clearness.*
Mohandas Gandhi

*It takes courage to demand time for yourself.
At first glance, it may seem to be the ultimate
in selfishness, a real slap in the face to those
who love and depend on you. It's not.
It means you care enough to want to see the
best in yourself and give only the best to others.*
Shale Paul

Key elements of mindfulness:

- ◆ Relaxation
- ◆ Being in the present
- ◆ Letting go of thoughts

There are plenty of ways to practice what some call meditation. You can do it deliberately while sitting in a classic meditation pose, by attending to your breathing in a yoga class, or simply by going into a "zone" while exercising or doing a simple task or by staring off into space. Letting go this way is useful for everyone. This Tip is about what you, as a nutrition therapist, can gain.

Benefits:

It's grounding for us. We are called on to be in empathetic resonance with people all day. When we are well grounded, we can slip into compassion more cleanly and then let go as each client leaves the office, creating room for us or for our next client. Many of our clients are anxious or stressed, and it's easy for us to pick this up. If we are practiced at letting go, we will be able to let go of this stress (that isn't ours anyway) more smoothly.

Mindfulness encourages us to **get into a creative or intuitive state.** In Tip #10, Reframing, I discuss putting clients' problems into a different context, allowing flexibility for change. Doing this requires a creative state of mind, one that is free-flowing and relaxed. Meditation promotes this state.

Meditation offers practice at focusing on **process rather than outcome.** Those who practice yoga know the feeling of simply doing the poses with no thought to what the benefit will be. Our focus during client sessions tends to be on the outcome we and our clients want. It can be useful at times to shift our focus to the process that is happening in the session or to the process the clients are describing in their lives. Meditation and yoga offer practice at making this shift.

Mindfulness supports **letting go of what we can't control.** There is much we can't control in our work. We can't *make* a young woman struggling with anorexia eat more. We can't *make* our clients keep appointments. When we let go of what we try to *make* happen, it's then clearer what we *can* do and it's easier to do it.

Meditation gives us **practice at letting go of our egos.** The more we get out of our own way during sessions, the more helpful we are to clients. We listen better when we are able to pause our own thoughts long enough to let in what the client is saying. This practice supports us to respond to our clients rather than react out of our own emotions.

140

Meditation (or yoga) may be the one sphere of our lives where there's **no judgment** or level of achievement; we just do what we can at whatever level of practice we are. We can choose to approach nutrition counseling without self-judgment. Mindfulness helps us be there with our clients with whatever level of expertise we possess.

We can **set an example for our clients**. Many of our clients are anxious or respond to stress by eating (or restricting food). If we suggest stress-management techniques to our clients, we can share that we care for ourselves this way as well.

Case Study: Meditation

A dietitian shared this personal experience:

> I hit a particularly hard time in my own therapy. I was reaching out to my therapist on the phone frequently for emotional support and regulation. The therapist set a boundary on this and told me to put some intention behind my self-care and emotional management. She suggested I meditate, journal, do yoga, etc. and if I needed to call in an EMERGENCY or wanted another appointment, that was no problem.
>
> So in my frustration and knowing this therapist was right, I set out to meditate every day for 20 to 30 minutes. I already had CDs from Jon Kabat-Zinn and a few others, so I set aside time daily to do it. I found my thought process slowing down and I started to see more choices in personal and professional dilemmas. I began to see the world more in Technicolor and be more mindful of all aspects of life. My marriage improved, and client sessions went better. Most notably, I felt more confident and better able to handle difficult clients and situations by RESPONDING and not REACTING.
>
> I have continued this regimen and have found it to be one of the most helpful aspects of practice. I now realize even more than before that one's personal state of tranquility has a lot to do with the dynamics that develop in a session. It frees the clients to be in their space more instead of tangling up in a mess of countertransference. As my therapist said, it helps with anxiety and reactivity, because you start to go from a 2 to a 4 instead of from a 6 to an 8 (on a 10-point anxiety scale)!

I knew that at some point my experience could benefit others, but during this growth spurt, I was struggling......sigh..... I'm so glad that I can share this with others.

Practice Steps: Incorporating Mindfulness

1. Do you already have some life practices that contribute to mindfulness? Find ways to practice them more consistently.
2. If you don't practice mindfulness yet, consider joining a yoga class or a mindfulness meditation class.
3. If a class doesn't work for you, set aside 10 to 30 minutes each day for sitting and letting go of your thoughts. Remember that there is no "right way" to do it. Letting go of thoughts does not mean that you don't have thoughts. Of course you do. Notice them and let them float away. It helps to have instruction at first, so check out these resources:

   Emotional Alchemy by Tara Bennett-Goleman

   The Power of Now by Eckhart Tolle

   Wherever You Go, There You Are by Jon Kabat-Zinn

   "Mindfulness Meditation" (recordings) by Jon Kabat-Zinn

4. Some people prefer to practice mindfulness as a part of their daily lives. Pick a few routine activities such as folding laundry or doing dishes and do them while fully focused on the present and the activity.
5. To practice using mindfulness to aid problem-solving, find a small problem you are struggling with. Set it aside and go to a yoga class or sit down and meditate without focusing on the problem. As you roll up your mat or end the meditation, bring the issue up again and notice how many more options have appeared.
6. For resources on mindful eating for you and your clients check out The Center for Mindful Eating at www.tcme.org.

My Experiments With Mindfulness

What I observe:

_____
_____
_____
_____
_____
_____
_____
_____
_____
_____
_____
_____
_____
_____
_____
_____
_____

How I will experiment:

_____
_____
_____
_____
_____
_____
_____
_____
_____
_____
_____
_____
_____
_____
_____
_____
_____

Tip #20
Unpacking Meaning

*Begin every day expecting to be
surprised and you will be.*

I am often asked for training on listening skills. We all know how important listening is, but **how is effective listening actually done?** This Tip provides more about the process of unpacking meaning that was mentioned in Tip #7, Assessing Readiness for Change.

You may have noticed that many people talk as if they are completely understood and everyone can read their minds. They don't fully explain what they are saying and **expect listeners to fill in the blanks.** Sometimes listeners mind-read accurately and sometimes they do not.

If you are going to help your client, an essential step is to **work to understand the client's meanings.** This works best when you hold the assumption that you don't understand what your client just said. This assumption allows you to uncover fascinating and important details.

Clues indicating you might need to unpack more meaning:

- Your client is stuck in the behavior-change process.
- You sense the client's resistance to change.
- You realize that you've been doing all the talking for a while.
- You hear something that sounds important to you.
- The client is arguing with you.
- You are puzzled and realize you may be proceeding with a mistaken understanding of what the client wants.

- You hear a generic word or phrase that could have several meanings, such as "I want to feel better" or "That doesn't work." (Do you know exactly what "that" refers to?)

What unpacking will do for you and your client:

- The client will feel heard and cared about.
- It quickly takes you out of the oppositional role and puts you solidly on the same side as your client. This is the first step in working with resistance.
- You avoid wasting time on goals that don't matter to the client.

Getting yourself ready:

To truly unpack your client's meaning, you must **make a shift**. For example, when you are in an "educating mode," most of the energy in the session is flowing from you to the client. This does not lend itself to being open to the client's input. You have an agenda and goals in mind. This stance has its place, but the stance that works for exploring meaning is quite the opposite.

The **ideal position is very open**, holding no agenda. You might want to find a word, an image, or a physical posture that symbolizes this open state for you. I find the word "curiosity" works for me. I also find that my eyes blink a lot and then are wide open as I settle into this mode. Knowing how this feels to you can help you shift into an open mode.

This isn't to say that an educating mode (or any other, for that matter) is wrong. The **skilled counselor can shift** stances easily during a session, adopting the most useful one for the particular moment.

Language To Transition into an Unpacking Mode:

- "I'm wondering. Would it be helpful to explore what this is all about for you?"
- "This sounds important. Would it be OK if we take a moment to understand this better so I can best help you?"
- "When I say ... I tend to mean ... Is that what you mean or is it different for you?"
- "What matters to you about ...?"
- "What does ... mean to you?"

Questions that continue the unpacking process:

- "And if you had ... what would that do for you?"
- "What are the best and worst parts?"
- "Would it help to talk more about that part?"
- "What matters most about it?"
- "Are there parts of this that mean more to you than others?"
- "Is this what matters the most to you or is there something else we're missing?"

Case Study: Unpacking Meaning

Robert called me for an appointment saying he needed to lose about 40 pounds because he has high blood pressure. He sounded intelligent and motivated.

A week later, at the first visit, I learned that he is a successful engineer who has lost and gained 40 pounds twice. This gave me a clue that he had conflicting intentions and that exploring more of what was important to him would be essential. I asked him, on a scale of 1 to 10, how important it was to him to lose weight. He surprised me by saying, "About a 3." I told him I was puzzled about this. He had called for the appointment in his busy schedule and come in to see me. It must have some importance to him. He said that he wasn't really worried about his blood pressure since it was controlled well with medication and that his clothes all fit well enough. He figured his knees might hurt less often if he weighed less, but this wasn't a big deal.

He then told me, with much feeling, that to his wife, his losing weight was an "11." He knew that she worried about his health and that it bothered her that he did not look as attractive as he had when they met 20 years ago. I asked what *was* important to him, if losing weight was not. He got a big smile and said that enjoying food was one of the most important things in his life. He almost giggled as he admitted being a "meat-and-potatoes guy." He looked forward to meals, especially ones with his family when there was time to sit and talk. When he was growing up, dinner was a comforting and pleasant time of day. He has two school-age children and loves to spend mealtimes with his family.

146

I smiled and repeated all this back to make sure I understood and to let him know that I heard him. I acknowledged that if we were going to work together, we would need to accept his love of food and work that into whatever changes we came up with. He seemed relieved that I accepted he didn't care about losing weight. He then told me that maybe it was about a "5" in importance that he lose weight since he did love his wife very much and didn't want to make her a widow anytime soon. I had learned some very important things about him in that first session. As we worked together, I kept in mind what really mattered to him and did not assume that weight loss was his most important goal.

Sample Dialog: Unpacking Meaning

This client was referred by her doctor. She is 45 years old, 5-foot-6 and 155 pounds.

Mary: I've got to get this weight off because now the doctor says I have diabetes.

Stop for a moment and notice your assumptions about this client. What will your goals be? What strategies will you use to get to those goals? What do you assume matters most to her?

Molly: So your doctor said you have diabetes, Mary. I'd like to find out more about your reaction to this news so I can best help you.

Mary: Well, he just said it's borderline, but that it could get worse if I don't lose weight.

Molly: So you want my help losing weight.

Mary: Only if I have to. I'm OK with my weight. I've always been this way. Most of the women in my family are much bigger. I think a size 14 is fine.

Molly: So you'd only be OK with losing weight if it helped your blood sugar.

Mary: I guess so. What I'm really upset about is my energy. I've been so tired recently. I usually have so much energy. That's the reason I went to the doctor and he did some tests and told me my blood sugar was up. He said that can make you tired. Is that right?

Molly: It sure can, and your energy can come right back as soon as your blood sugar is normal. So what matters most to you is your energy. Could you tell me more about that?

Mary: Yes, I am a teacher and love my work. I want to be able to keep up with the kids. And I have two good friends whom I love to travel with. We take a big trip in the summer and a shorter one at spring break. We love seeing new places, and I would hate to run out of energy on the trips.

Molly: So your main goal is feeling better and having energy. There certainly are things you can do to quickly bring your blood sugar in the normal range before we even think about weight loss. Shall we try them first?

Mary: That sounds great!

Molly: What else is important to you?

Mary: Well, is there a way we could work on my stamina, too? I don't know if diabetes affects that, but I have sometimes wished on our trips that I could walk for longer. At so many fun places you need to walk a lot.

Molly: Oh, that goal fits right in here! The very best way to increase your stamina for walking is to build up slowly now, well before the trip. And it turns out that walking is really good for your blood sugar.

Mary: So I can be doing two things at once? I have always thought I should get more exercise. Let's work on that.

Molly: Yes, we can focus on what the walking will do for your stamina on trips and you will get the side benefit of better blood sugar. We can also look at how you are eating. I'm sure we can find some simple changes that will have an immediate effect on your blood sugar.

Mary: OK, because I really am sick of being so tired all the time.

Practice Steps: Advancing Your Unpacking Skills

1. Work to adopt a "clueless" stance. There are important things you don't know about your client's meaning. This is ALWAYS true, even when the client says something very straightforward that you have heard from clients before.   There is always *something* that you missed or that the client hasn't quite figured out yet. If you find quotes helpful, place the one at the beginning of this Tip on your desk or in some client charts.

2. Go into your next session with the above belief solidly in place. Search for opportunities to get curious. Sometimes it's just a word you hear that could have various meanings or it may be something the client says with emphasis.

3. Take a deep breath (or anything else that will help you shift) and go into curiosity mode.

4. Use the unpacking questions over and over.

5. As you hear meanings from your client, repeat them back in your own words and ask if you've heard them right. (See Tip #6, Mirroring.)

6. Stick with being the curiosity machine for as long as you and your client can bear it.

7. Do a final summary of what was unpacked and check with your client to make sure you got all the important points.

8. If you think this client is game, ask if it was OK that you got so curious. Ask if it helped in any way. If the answer is "yes," you could unpack that (i.e., *how* exactly did it help?).

9. Later in supervision or in a quiet moment, review how the process went. What did you learn that you'd like to apply again? What didn't work? What do you need more practice doing?

10. Use what you learned in this exercise to revise your unpacking style and practice with the next client.

My Experiments With Unpacking Meaning

What I observe:

_____
_____
_____
_____
_____
_____
_____
_____
_____
_____
_____
_____
_____
_____
_____
_____
_____

How I will experiment:

_____
_____
_____
_____
_____
_____
_____
_____
_____
_____
_____
_____
_____
_____
_____
_____
_____
_____

Tip #21
Time Boundaries in Sessions

Good fences make good neighbors.
Robert Frost

We are what we repeatedly do.
Excellence, then, is not an act, but a habit.
Aristotle

Careful tending of time limits in nutrition sessions is one of the many ways to **set appropriate professional boundaries**. Other areas for setting limits (covered in other Tips) are deciding what to disclose about yourself, limiting topics to nutrition, responding to missed appointments and cancellations, insisting clients work with a therapist if they need it, and handling dual relationships. Many of the concepts here can be applied to other limits on your professional time, such as the length of phone calls and use of e-mail.

Some clients seem to understand time limits naturally, and **some will always push** them. All clients need us to guard the edges. A general rule of thumb: Clients who push your time limits are the ones who benefit the most from your firm application of limits and they will never acknowledge it or thank you.

Why time limits are important:

- The **next client** on your schedule may be annoyed if you start late.
- You may become **resentful** and therefore not as available to this client and others.
- If you don't get that 5 minutes to go to the bathroom, take a deep breath and/or jot some notes, you will **burn out.**
- Careful tending of time limits reminds you and the client that **all professional boundaries** are important. Time boundaries are just the most obvious.
- You convey that your time (and the client's) is **valuable.**
- Most clients are more comfortable if they know what to expect, so you are **doing them a service** by keeping the time consistent.

Common obstacles to keeping session time limits:

- Are you **scheduling** clients appropriately? For example, is it realistic for you to complete a first visit and be ready to move on to the next one in 60 minutes? Depending on your setting, this may be quite realistic. Or it may be expecting too much. For follow-up sessions, some clients may need longer than others. Can you plan for that and bill accordingly?
- If you see clients in your home, would switching to a **professional office** help you? A home contributes to a sense of being on "social time," which is usually open-ended.
- What **expectations** do the clients have before the first session? Do you or your assistant convey professional time limits on the phone? If you work in a doctor's office or gym, is others' sense of time affecting your work?
- What pressures are you putting on yourself? Do you wonder if you have given your clients enough for today? **What is enough?** How to measure whether you have made your fee? Basically, you can't. You do your best. It is up to clients to decide whether you are worth their time and money. What are they paying you for? So many pounds lost? Symptom relief? Or are they paying you for your time and for you to do your very best to address their goals during the time allotted?
- Are you avoiding the end of the session because that is when you ask for **the fee?**
- If there are particular clients you always let stay longer, what is it about them you are responding to? For example, is the **client's**

anxiety hooking you in to trying harder? (See Tip #5, How to Respond to Your Client's Strong Feelings, and Tip #15, Staying on Topic.)

♦ Are you letting clients stay longer so they will like you? Clients are not here to meet **your need to be liked**. Until it's truly time to end with a client because the goals have been achieved, expect that something will always be incomplete in each session. How are you going to get a client to come back if you meet all the needs in a single session?

How to ease the process:

♦ **Set expectations** on the phone and at the beginning of each session. "Let's see, we have 50 minutes, so what would you like to focus on today?" This assumes you may not get to all of what the client needs that day.

♦ Position a **clock** clearly visible to the client and another one for you.

♦ If the client comes in **late**: "I'm afraid I have a client scheduled right after you, so I can't offer to give you the full session time. We need to end at 2:50." If you are able and willing to give the full time, make it clear that it will not always be so.

♦ **Mention the time** at certain intervals: "I see we have 10 minutes left. Are we addressing what you need today?" This is particularly important with clients who push your limits.

♦ With some, you may need to **hit them over the head** by asking for the payment, scheduling the next visit, or getting up and walking to the door.

♦ If you schedule your own appointments, **look for signs** during the initial phone call that this client will push time limits. Then, be sure to discuss time at the beginning of the session and periodically.

♦ For home offices, what can you do to make your home feel to you and to the client like an office? Put a sign outside and refer to your "office" even if it is also your den. Use language that makes it clear you are on **"professional time."** Use phrases such as "your session time," "your 50 minutes," "my office hours."

♦ Some clients will respond to **empathy**. "I know it's hard to stop. This is all so important to you." "Holding it until next week may be hard, but remember that real change happens slowly."

♦ If **collecting the fee** is hard for you, set a policy of collecting it at the beginning.

♦ Promising to **pick up the same topic** at the next session may ease the end of the current one. Make a note so you can keep your promise.

♦ If you are working behaviorally with a client and need to **end with specific plans**, attend to moving along earlier in the session. For example, you may need to say, "Well, we have only 10 minutes left. Let's make sure you have your plan in place for this week."

It's not easy to **examine your own process** critically. You may need the help of a colleague, supervisor or life coach. For example, having unrealistic expectations is almost impossible to notice by yourself.

Someone else can help you find a **few key phrases** to keep in mind at the beginning and at critical points during sessions. For example: "I'd really like to meet all her needs today, but I can only do so much." "It's in the client's best interest to end on time." Design phrases that specifically address your stuck places.

Question **other professionals** about how they manage to slip into their professional selves during sessions.

You might **consider psychotherapy** if insecurity about your competence or your need to be liked gets in the way of ending sessions on time.

Case Study: A Supervision Session on Time Boundaries

Molly: On our last supervision call, we were on a very interesting topic and I needed to cut it off because the hour was up. I want to ask all of you what that was like for you since you were then in the same position that our clients are when we have to cut off sessions.

Suzanne Girard Eberle, MS, RD: I guess I'm used to it, so I don't personalize it as much as I imagine my clients do. At the same time I'm thinking, wow, *I* don't want to do what you did.

Molly: That is really the point, Suzanne, because my guess is our clients *can* get used to it. The first time, they might not. They might have trouble taking care of themselves and realizing it's not personal. They *can* get used to it. That doesn't mean they like it. It's not wonderful, but they don't have a choice. Anybody else have any reactions?

Robin Millet, MS, RD, CDN: When I have to end a session if we're in the middle of something important like what happened on our supervision call, it feels like we lost momentum on a really interesting topic. Can you get it back if you need to in the next session? You can write notes to be sure that you follow up on the topic, but it is different because you're not in the heat of the discussion.

Molly: Exactly. And that is a concern that you run into with your clients. You worry about that, do you?

Robin: Yes, for my clients but also for myself. *I will miss discovering something really important if I don't have the opportunity to sort of delve into it right then.*

Molly: Right. It is a loss, isn't it? It's a potential loss. None of us welcome losing something we believe will be of value.

Gale Welter, MS, RD, CSCS: On the last call, I just took it as, "OK, that's the way it is," and I've had enough of my own therapy to know that happens all the time. But I will say I feel worse when I'm the person that has to cut it off. Especially knowing we didn't really get to the point the person expected even if we got to some other valuable stuff. It's hard when I know they didn't get what they came in the door expecting to get and may have not wanted to leave without. But I am getting better at follow-up. I used to work expecting to have only one session with them. Now I'm empowered somewhere near the half-hour mark to talk about how we can handle some of these things that have come up. I set the stage for multiple appointments.

Molly: Gale, I don't want to lose something that you just said that sounds important. In your experience, when you're on the client's end, it's not as hard as when you are the one reminding about time and cutting it off.

Suzanne: Yes! Especially since they're paying money and they have this set of expectations. I'm pretty generous with my time and then when I do reel it in, it's amazing to me the ones that feel like I'm now cutting them off.

Molly: Of course, if you set a precedent for going over, they're more likely to feel disappointed when you try to do something different. It's a lot like being a parent. If you let a kid get away with something several times, you are more apt to get a tantrum when you hold the line.

Suzanne: I'm trying to be really conscious when I get a new client. I'm going to end these on time because I want to get off on the right foot.

Molly: To a large extent, Gale is absolutely right that it's harder on us than it is on them. There may indeed be clients who are disappointed and sad and they go away feeling some disappointment. I doubt it lasts very long. If they're severely disappointed and totally thrown off by it that may be a clue to a personality disorder. (That's a discussion for another time.) Generally, people cope because they know that this is what happens in the world. There *are* limits, and if they haven't completely figured that out yet, you can help them figure out that they're not always going to get what they want. If this is one of the primary lessons your client still needs to learn, this is more the therapist's job than yours. But you can be one of the people that helps the client with it. As Gale pointed out, most of it is our stuff. I experience this, too. "Oh, I haven't given her all she needs!" Is that what you're feeling, Suzanne? "I haven't done my job or I haven't given her enough for her money."

Suzanne: Yes, especially in my private practice. I've heard clients say about other RDs, "I didn't get anything from seeing her; it was a total waste of time." I hear this and I worry they will say this about me.

Molly: There are people who either are impossible to please or they want something that is unrealistic. Or maybe what you do best does not happen to be what they need.

Suzanne: Molly, it would help me to understand from a counseling perspective what is detrimental about letting sessions go on. I enjoy that I'm this person they feel they can talk to, so I could use some things to keep in mind about this giving lots of time not being 100 percent helpful.

Molly: Thank you for asking for what you need. Let's look at the practical aspects. If you let it go an hour and 20 minutes a few times in a row because you don't happen to have a client right afterwards and then the next time you do have a client right afterwards or you have an appointment for yourself. Then it's a whole lot harder on you and the client, isn't it? It can feel like you're taking away something that the client had before. Again, it's like being a parent. You're firm on the times that you really could give in so that it's easy later.

Let's look at it from another perspective. I heard a story awhile ago that totally floored me, and I haven't forgotten it. A new therapy client came in, and as usual I asked her about past therapy experiences. She told me of her first experience of therapy with a family therapist that she saw with her husband. He was warm and giving and helpful, but it began to bother her that he would go way over an hour. Nothing was said about time at all. She saw two problems from her perspective. One was that her session often started really late because he went over with the person before. But more importantly, she had this sense of not knowing when it was going to end. She wasn't sure whether she should open up a new topic because she didn't know whether he would go on longer or not. It had an unbounded feel that felt increasingly uncomfortable and caused her to pull back from the openness she had first felt. She needed the time boundaries in order to feel safe enough to open up and work. Her story has been a lesson to me. She got less value from the experience even though she got a lot of time for her money. Does that make sense to you, Suzanne?

Suzanne: Yes, I'm just trying to remind myself that this can't all be positive, otherwise we'd all have these run-on sessions and everyone would be getting fixed really well.

Molly: There is another value to keeping time boundaries. For some of our clients, ending a meal is problematic. The moment when "I've had enough and it's time to end even though there's some delicious-looking food on the plate." Well, ending a session is an awful lot like that, isn't it? They get a taste, get some of what they need, and then, it's time to move on, and there will be another meal later. There'll be another session a few weeks later. Helping the client wrap it up and keep that boundary can help them with the process in ending a meal. Learning to say, "Well, I guess I'll pack up the food," is parallel to saying, "We'll end for now and this is the topic we will begin with next visit." Working on one moves the other along.

Gale: Do you ever share that with them?

Molly: Yes, occasionally. Especially with a client I've seen several times and there is a theme of meal endings being tough. I might point out, "You know this ending of sessions is tricky, too, isn't it?" Or I might not. It depends on how much insight the person has.

Gale: Molly, I have thought of this before but I am not a person who likes to end things. I don't like to transition between one thing and another. If I'm home, it's a pain getting to work. If I'm at work, it's a pain getting home. If I'm with someone, it's a pain getting to the next person. If I'm eating my own dinner, I don't like to end eating. I've never looked at it this way before, but it's a lot of my own lack of edges. It may be a way of relaxing because I don't have a lot of downtime. I think it is a rebellion in my later life from twenty-some years of definite scheduling with kids and husband and everything working like clockwork. Now I can spread out, but I overshoot it.

Molly: Are there ways, Gale, for you to take care of yourself, acknowledging that downtime is important to you so you don't have to do it in your business?

Gale: So that's the part that is "my stuff." Also, I can find the value of ending so that I am on time for the next client, and I have time to write up notes. I'm constantly catching up or running to my next appointment across campus like I did yesterday because I let this young lady talk me over.

Molly: It's not easy to cut people off when they want to keep going, is it? By the way, I'll share with you all that two weeks ago, when it was time to end our call, I believe I said I had a client out in my waiting room. I actually didn't have a client. I decided to deliberately use that partly for my benefit, to give me an excuse. That may be cowardice on my part, but it helped me stay firm. For a while, you may need something to support you like looking at the clock and saying, "There's a conference call I have to get onto at 11."

Suzanne: I've had my husband call at a certain time.

Kathee Varner, RD: I've literally had to stand up with clients who were sitting down and head towards the door. I think it's important that we as professionals model those boundaries because that's what we're trying to teach them with their eating problems.

Also, see case study of Karl on page 121.

Practice Steps: Tightening Up Time Boundaries

1. Do you frequently go over the time you plan for sessions? If so, first determine if this is a problem you want to address. Look at the list of reasons that time limits might be important. If none of these are important to you, you can stop here and move on to Tip #22.
2. If you decide to work on staying on schedule, examine the whole process so you can pinpoint what needs to shift. Which common obstacles listed above might be true in your situation?
3. Pick one or a few strategies suggested in the Tip and experiment.
4. If you continue to struggle, talk it over with a colleague or seek supervision.

My Experiments With Time Boundaries

What I observe:

_____
_____
_____
_____
_____
_____
_____

How I will experiment:

_____
_____
_____
_____
_____
_____
_____

Tip #22
Detecting and Avoiding Burnout

*The great advantage of being in a rut is that when
one is in a rut, one knows exactly where one is.*
Arnold Bennett

*When we are motivated by goals that have deep meaning,
by dreams that need completion, by pure love
that needs expressing, then we truly live life.*
Greg Anderson

Here are some clues you may headed for burnout:

- Feeling exhausted often
- Fantasizing about being somewhere else or having a different career or job
- Feeling bored
- Getting cynical, losing your sense of humor
- Feeling incompetent, ineffective, beating yourself up
- Dreading going to work, feeling relieved when leaving
- Not caring the way you used to about the patients or your field
- Avoiding the work, procrastinating, avoiding patients
- Spending all your waking hours working
- Irritability with those close to you (If you listen, loved ones will tip you off to burnout.)

Burnout happens when you do not have **the support you need** to do the level of work you are doing. If enough of the needs that matter to you are met, you don't burn out.   Some needs are more important to you than

160

others. Notice which ones are key for you so you can adjust your life to address them:

- **Appreciation:** We all need our world to tell us that we are of value. The more approval and gratitude we get, the less likely we will burn out. If you need lots of appreciation, that's OK. You can choose to support your world to give you more. When those around you spontaneously give you positive feedback, thank them and tell them how much it means to you. Remind them to provide it whenever they feel like it. Keep a file of thank-you notes from clients.

- **Breaks:** Vacations, days or parts of days off. (These could be weekly, monthly or spontaneous.) What kinds of breaks work best for you? Getting this need met might mean tweaking your weekly or daily schedule to allow for regular breaks.

- **Community:** The sense that you are not in this alone. It's people to turn to for advice, perspective and empathy.   What kind of community do you need for each kind of work you do? Be sure to include parenting work and your hobbies as well as your job. In private practice, there is a tendency to isolate. Do you need a regular meeting time with peers? If you are the only dietitian in your setting, do you need to find others doing similar work and get together on a regular basis?

- **Control:** A certain degree of control over your life is essential to avoid burnout. If this is an issue for you right now, first acknowledge what you do and don't have control over.   To cope with what is not in your control, see Tip #19, How a Mindfulness Practice Aids Our Work. Start working to change what you can. For example, is a flex-time schedule a possibility? You'll never know if you don't ask.

- **Collaboration:** Bouncing ideas off others can be an energizing experience, especially if you work alone. Adding more brainstorming with others may reduce your sense of burnout.

- **Diversification:** This can mean a variety of duties in your full-time job, making time for serious hobbies, or splitting into two jobs or careers. For example, a friend who is a nurse struggled with burnout for years before she finally switched to part time and also became a part-time real estate agent. She got to continue nursing (a career she still loves) while expanding into another of her interests.

- **Excitement/Passion:** Know what compels you and go for it. If what pulled you into the field is still exciting (working with kids, being around food, teaching, helping people have better lives, or whatever), clarify what that passion is and work to find ways to live it out at this stage in your career.

- ◆ **Growth Edge/Challenge:** A common cause of burnout is work that is too familiar and easy. If you feel you can do your job "with your eyes closed," find a way to stretch yourself: a new skill, or computer program, a new disease to learn more about, a new population to work with, public speaking, etc.
- ◆ **Gratitude:** If you find yourself complaining a lot, add a gratitude routine to your life and see what happens. We all have things we are grateful for. We just forget to notice them. You could start a list and add a new one every evening.
- ◆ **Humor:** Search for the fun in whatever you do. Humor goes a long way toward lightening the tough parts of life.
- ◆ **Variety:** If you are often bored, try doing routine things differently. Drive a different route to work, experiment with different snacks or meals, do your job duties in a different order. These may not work for everyone, but give it a try.

It's tempting to chuck it all when you feel burned out. This might mean quitting your job or even the whole field. Before you do something so drastic, it's wise to **see if you can tweak things** instead. You may be surprised at how much better you feel when you slowly work at getting your needs met where you are. If you've worked at it for a while and hit too many brick walls, then it may be time to look elsewhere. At least then you will know you gave it a good try.

Finally, **don't do it alone!** Trying to fight burnout alone is like trying to climb out of a deep pit with no one throwing you a rope.

Case Study: One Dietitian's Journey Through Burnout

Carol Nocella, RD, CDN, of Bayside, N.Y., sent me this story:

> I have been an RD for about seven years. I have experienced burnout several times. I look back on my story now as a process of struggling to find my niche in this field. After becoming an RD, I started work at a hospital clinical job. I found it very unsatisfying because of the short stays. The patients were in and out so fast, and they really didn't care about diet education. The doctors at this particular hospital also didn't care about the dietitians, so it was very frustrating.

I moved on to a nursing home thinking that long-term stays would equal job satisfaction, since I would be getting to know the patients. I eventually worked my way up to chief clinical dietitian, but the stress was ridiculous! I found all the "rules and regulations" of the Department of Health and JCAHO regarding strict documentation guidelines were just that -- strict and rigid. While I agree that documentation is extremely important and I am a stickler for it, I found I was spending the majority of my time writing "perfect" notes and not enough time with the patients. I also found our "interdisciplinary team" (speech, OT, PT, nursing, recreation, etc.) were all working separately and not as a team. Everyone tried to blame everyone else for his own mistakes.

So, against everyone's advice, I made the big move to quit and became a fee-for-service dietitian. I contract with several agencies. I did it slowly and "weaned myself" from the full-time position. At first, I worked full time and took side jobs in the early evening: private practice, group homes, and home care. I then cut back to three days a week at the nursing home, and once my side jobs built up, I quit the nursing home altogether.

I now work in different settings every day. I rent space at a wellness center and do some private practice. I work one day a week at a rehab facility for teens. I do some home-care visits and work in several group homes for the mentally retarded doing nutrition counseling, staff education and menu planning.

I am a much happier person and have finally beaten the insomnia and fatigue. It was a risky move at the time because my husband was laid off from work, but I followed my intuition and it has worked out favorably! I believe my health comes first. I know this is not for everyone as it means giving up paid vacations, paid holidays and sick days as well as medical coverage. There are so many different areas and ways to work as a dietitian; you just have to find the right one. I believe taking the risk of change was worth it. And if what I'm doing now stops working for me, I can always find something else. Writing this down was therapeutic and it made me feel better about what I have been able to accomplish by taking risks!

Practice Steps: Problem-Solving Burnout

1. Are you at risk for burnout? Use the checklist above to look for the signs.
2. Use the list of needs to pinpoint the areas that are problematic for you.
3. Search for ways to alter your life to support you better. Make one or two changes at a time and assess again.
4. Remember, it works much better to do this process with support. Talk with colleagues, family members and friends and/or find a life coach.
5. Make this tweaking process a routine part of your life!

My Experiments With Burnout

What I observe:

_____
_____
_____
_____
_____
_____
_____
_____
_____

How I will experiment:

_____
_____
_____
_____
_____
_____
_____
_____
_____

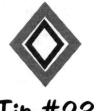

Tip #23
Triangulation

Blame is demeaning;
responsibility is empowering.
Victoria Moran

Praise and blame
gain and loss
pleasure and sorrow
come and go like the wind.
To be happy, rest like a great tree
in the midst of them all.
The Buddha

When **two people are in conflict,** there is a tendency for one or both to involve another person. It seems as if this makes it easier to handle or resolve the conflict. It doesn't. In the short run, triangulation may be effective in reducing anxiety. For example, when it feels unacceptable or unsafe to express anger or confront differences with a particular person, the relationship can remain fairly stable and calm on the surface if the angry person acts angry with someone with whom the person feels safe. However, in the long run, it does not work because the real conflict is not addressed. Triangulation distracts from the real conflict and its resolution. This displacement also harms the second relationship. Some triangles exist briefly while others are long-standing and rigid.

This process of triangulation is extremely common and **part of human nature.** That doesn't mean it's healthy or effective. When we, as professionals, get pulled into a conflict, our work is compromised.

Examples of triangulation you may see in your work:

- A client who is in conflict with the therapist, parent or spouse **may ask you to intervene.**
- In families with unresolved conflict between the parents (or other family members), **a child may be triangulated.** If the child has an eating disorder, it can intensify the triangulation. The family attention is on the eating disorder and therefore distracted from the uncomfortable marital conflict.
- A parent who is trying to get a child to eat more (or less) will **beg you to fix it** (for example, pull you into the conflict). This makes it hard for you to work directly with the child on the child's nutrition goals.
- A client struggling with an eating disorder may triangulate you into the conflict between the **two parts of the client's self.** You may be asked to side only with the eating-disorder side or only with the side that wants to recover. When you stay fully in contact with both sides, you are more effective in guiding your client to recovery.

Clues that triangulation may be occurring:

- You feel **tempted** to jump into a conflict that does not directly involve you.
- Your **client tells you things** that would best be said directly to her parents or therapist.
- You sense anxiety or emotional energy in the room and find yourself **puzzled** that it seems misplaced or irrational.

How to avoid being pulled into a conflict (and how to get out):

- **Stay calm:** Use a low-key voice tone and language. Mirror the distress you hear (see Tip #6) without adding to the energy you are sensing.
- **Stay out** (if it's not your fight): Refuse to get in the middle, blame, fix or take sides. Stay clear about what the core conflicts are. When asked to intervene, support the person to address the conflict directly and not through you.

♦ **Stay there:** Stay present in the relationship (or relationships). Though it may be tempting to side with one person, stay in contact with each person. If you have a conflict with someone, address it directly.

These techniques work to avoid being pulled into someone else's conflict. They also are effective to **avoid initiating a triangulation process** yourself. When there is a real difference of opinion or conflict between you and your client (or a parent or a therapist), acknowledge it. Clarify what that conflict is and work to resolve it directly with the person you differ with. If you suspect triangulation and can't easily locate an original conflict that is being redirected, consult with the client's therapist or seek supervision.

Long-standing, rigid family triangulation patterns occur frequently, especially in families that have someone with an eating disorder. It is **not your job** to resolve them. That's the work of family therapy. You can support that work, however, by refusing to be pulled in, by staying in close contact with the therapist, and by encouraging the family to engage in therapy.

Case Study: Triangulation in Teen Weight Management

I got a call from Tracy's mother, Ann, asking for an appointment. She said that Tracy, 14, had been gaining weight for the last year and wanted to see a nutritionist. I asked Ann if this was Tracy's idea and she assured me it was. I told her that we would do the beginning of the initial session with both Ann and Tracy, but the majority of the time, I would likely want to meet with only Tracy.

Tracy was a pleasant girl who appeared, at most, 10 percent above ideal weight. Ann went on at length about how Tracy had always been such a "cute little string bean of a girl" and that she had been telling her daughter for months that if she didn't start paying attention, she would get really fat. Tracy rolled her eyes and said very little as her mother went on about how Tracy really needed to change her eating habits. I asked Ann to go to the waiting room. As she left, she listed several specific things she wanted me to tell Tracy "because maybe she will listen to you."

Ann had set me up to be on her side and to get right into the battle she was having with Tracy. I made a point of not picking up Ann's side by first remaining quiet for a few moments and then asking Tracy for her response to what her mother had said. After a sigh, she said, "She does this all the time. She makes such a big deal about looks. I know she was a beauty queen and all that when she was my age, but I really don't care." I asked her how she felt about her weight. She said that at first she didn't like getting bigger. She was used to being one of the smallest in her class, so it seemed weird. I carefully asked about teasing or comments about her body by classmates or family members. Many teens will not share painful comments because of shame. She mentioned one comment with a smile, saying it was by a "stupid boy who thinks he likes me."

She soon began to talk about sports. She had recently discovered that her size helped in sports. "Don't tell Mom this, but I really think being a little heavier is better for soccer. I've been lifting weights in the gym at school and I think my legs are getting stronger. My aunt is a tennis player and she says I could be a good athlete." As soon as I heard "Don't tell Mom this," I knew that each side was trying to draw me into a conflict and I would need to work carefully to avoid this. By the end of the time with Tracy, we had agreed to have a few sessions focusing on sports nutrition since she had no interest in losing weight. I invited Ann back in and asked Tracy to tell her mother our agreement. She asked me to tell her. I reluctantly agreed. Checking to gain Tracy's agreement on each sentence, I told Ann what the two of us would do over the next few sessions. To my surprise, Ann seemed fine with this.

After two more sessions with Tracy alone, I got an upset voice message from Ann. Tracy had just had an annual doctor's visit and her weight had not gone down. Ann accused me of "not doing any good." She again listed specific things she wanted me to tell Tracy, such as what to eat in the lunchroom at school and not to stop for snacks on the way home. She said that at the first session she thought that I was humoring Tracy by talking about sports and that I really agreed with her that she needed to lose weight. It was time for me to work on my relationship with Ann. Since I knew that the conversation would not be short, I asked her to schedule a time to come in by herself. Ann began with all her complaints about Tracy's eating habits and even threw in a few other typical annoying teen behaviors unrelated to food. I listened only long enough to get a sense of a classic teen/mother conflict and then cut it off. I said, "I'm not the one who needs to hear all this. You two seem to have a lot of the typical mother/teen daughter conflicts. It is difficult to be the mother of such an active, bright girl. Have you considered getting some guidance?" I then told her about an educational program for parents of teens taught by a local family therapist. She agreed to look into it. Several more times during the session, Ann began to complain about Tracy and I cut her off again, thereby refusing to be pulled into the conflict. I asked whether she was willing to continue to allow me to work with Tracy on sports nutrition if Tracy wanted to. I brought this up quite deliberately because I wanted to show Ann that I had a working relationship with Tracy and ask for her support. She agreed. I also asked Ann to tell Tracy about her phone call and our meeting.

When I next saw Tracy, I asked her if her mother had told her about calling me. She said, "Yeah, she does that kind of thing all the time. I'm used to it." She didn't seem to want to talk about it more, so we moved on. Several times, Tracy told me things her mother said and complained that "she gets in my business too much." It was tempting to jump in and get on her side (I found Ann intrusive, too). Tracy even asked me to tell her mother to back off. I knew that would be jumping into the conflict, so instead I urged her to talk with her mother herself. When she told me things she didn't seem to be telling her mother, such as how much sports meant to her, I suggested she bring that up, but didn't push it. I saw Tracy about five times and then ended. A few years later, she called and wanted to meet once before going to college. She had an athletic scholarship and wanted some advice on eating well at school. I sensed a much improved mother/daughter relationship.

Fortunately, this family seems to have moved through the teen years relatively successfully. This illustrates how a normal developmental conflict can easily become about food and weight. It is common, as a nutrition professional, to experience pressure to get into such a conflict. It never helps to. In this family, there may have been another layer of triangulation such as a conflict between Ann and her husband or her own mother that she was trying to deal with by fighting with Tracy. Or, the energy on Ann's side of the conflict may have had more to do with her own body and weight concerns. This would be projection. (See Tip #14.) This is all speculation on my part. I was not their family therapist, so all I could do was address the nutrition concerns as well as I could while attempting to avoid being dragged into the family conflict.

Practice Steps: Triangulation

1. The next time you suspect triangulation, find some time to sit quietly and analyze it.
2. Search for the original conflict. Who are the primary people in conflict with each other? What is the conflict about? (You might not have a full answer.) It may be useful to diagram it. Show the two in conflict connected by a jagged line and show the line connecting the person being pulled into the conflict. Which person is pulling the third in? Or is the third jumping in unasked? Keep this diagram in your head as you proceed.
3. If you are being pulled into someone else's conflict, remind yourself that it is not your fight. Maintain a relationship with each person (even if it's difficult). Find calm, factual phrases to use with each of the people to maintain your distance.
4. If you are in conflict with someone and tempted to bring in a third party, take some time to calm down. Clarify exactly what the conflict is and what you can do to address it directly with the original person.
5. If a person you are in conflict with keeps trying to pull in someone else, make a request to discuss it one-on-one. Prepare by reminding yourself what matters to you and what it is you most want or need.

My Experiments With Triangulation

What I observe:

_____
_____
_____
_____
_____
_____
_____
_____
_____
_____
_____
_____
_____
_____
_____
_____

How I will experiment:

_____
_____
_____
_____
_____
_____
_____
_____
_____
_____
_____
_____
_____
_____
_____
_____
_____

Tip #24
Clients Who Don't Return

I wanted a perfect ending. Now I've learned, the hard way, that some poems don't rhyme, and some stories don't have a clear beginning, middle, and end.
Gilda Radner

*Do what you can,
with what you have
where you are.*
Theodore Roosevelt

Clients don't return for scheduled appointments for countless reasons:

- ◆ They are not ready to make the changes you suggest.
- ◆ They are in denial about having a condition that is best treated by lifestyle change.
- ◆ It's inconvenient to get to appointments.
- ◆ They are avoiding the discomfort and anxiety they believe the changes will bring.
- ◆ Their spouse, parent or boss thinks it's stupid, or a waste of time or money.
- ◆ They don't have the money for your fee and are too embarrassed to say so.
- ◆ Their neighbor handed them a diet book and they decided to try that instead.

... and this is only a small sample.

If the client doesn't return or call, you don't have enough information to know for sure why the treatment ended. Since human minds aren't comfortable with not knowing, you tend to speculate. This can be a fun exercise, but it's important to remember that it is less about truth than about trying to feel more comfortable.

Every now and then, you may get a chance to find out what happened with a client who comes back much later. This is a wonderful opportunity to get curious. You may be surprised at the answers. You will glean valuable information for your work with this client. For example, if the client says she wasn't ready, that is a clue to closely track her readiness for any changes this time. (See Tip #7.)

Should you follow up with clients who disappear? Questions to ask yourself:

- **How long** have you been seeing the client? If it's been only a visit or two, you may not have the rapport that warrants follow-up.
- What **agreement and/or contract** do you have? If you had a clear agreement to meet a certain number of times or the client has paid up front, you might consider calling to make sure the client knows your policy. If you had an agreement to work until specific health goals were met, you may choose to call or write as a reminder that the goals have not been met.
- Is there a **medical or ethical imperative** to follow up? Do you suspect the client is in denial about the seriousness of the condition or the need for treatment? If your professional belief is that the client needs to be in treatment, say it simply and clearly either by phone or in writing. If you are concerned about liability, a letter to the client with a copy to the doctor is wise.
- Are you following up because you can't stand the uncertainty or need the money the visits provide? **Get clear about your reasons** by talking it over with someone. If the reasons are about you, there are better ways to address them. For example, you can target your practice to those with whom you work best. If it's discomfort with what you can't control, try yoga, relaxation techniques or spiritual practices.

If you do follow up:

- State clearly and compassionately **what you know to be true**. For example, "Your blood sugar is still in a range that causes the complications we talked about." "I know that this work to recover from your eating disorder is scary for you."
- State what you believe is the **appropriate treatment**. For example, "It takes many months with ongoing support to make the lifestyle changes we talked about." "Giving up binging takes lots of steps and weekly visits work best."
- **Stay curious** and leave the door open to future work.
- **Offer what you can do** if the client returns.
- Respect the **client's choice**.

By the way, from a **marketing perspective**, it's a good idea to keep the contact information for all past clients so if you move or offer a new service, you can send out an announcement. This may prompt a few clients who are ready to come back.

Do you **want more of your clients to come back** for multiple visits? Do you believe they would benefit and you have more to provide? Even though many of the reasons are within the client, you may be able to increase your return rate if you examine how you conduct the first few visits. Attend to the process of building rapport. Include techniques of unpacking (Tip #20) and mirroring (Tip #6) to make sure you understand the client's goals and to communicate empathy. Explore what is important to the client and his confidence to change (Tip #7).

If you realize belatedly that you did not adequately listen to what the client wanted or pushed changes he wasn't ready for, take a moment to **forgive yourself for being human**. Beating yourself up does not contribute to progress in your counseling skills. You could choose to use this experience as an incentive to go back and practice some of the basics mentioned above with your next few clients.

It's helpful to examine **your reaction** to the client's not returning. First, notice the temptation to personalize it. Your mind may take the blame to try to gain a sense of control over something over which you have little control. It's rarely about you or something you did or didn't do. Most likely it is something that would surprise you.

A common reaction is annoyance. If the client doesn't show for a scheduled appointment, you lose that hour. It is also normal to react with concern. You may care about the client's health and are concerned that not all the necessary changes have been made. You may have the sense of **threads left hanging**. Especially with a client you saw for a long time, you never hear the end of the story and that is disconcerting. Care for yourself by talking with someone about it and finding ways to let go.

Case Study: A Client Who Cancels Appointments

Lauren Balkin, MS, RD, CDN, of New York City, sent this query to the Nutrition Entrepreneurs Listserv:

> I have a morbidly obese client whom I have been seeing for about nine months now. She understands my 24-hour cancellation policy, and I had to charge her once for not canceling before the 24 hours. She understood perfectly. We have a standing appointment every Thursday at 6:30, a very popular time slot as all of you could probably understand. The problem is this: She cancels 24 hours ahead of time probably eight out of 10 Thursdays. It is becoming a problem because, although it is 24 hours ahead of time, I lose out on that hour that I am seeing anyone. I try to call people to fill that slot, but by that time, they have already arranged another time to see me (I have extended my evening hours because of this) and worked their schedule around it. I understand that with morbidly obese people there are sometimes other issues with responsibility and commitment, but this is getting to be too much for me. I have gone above and beyond to help this client and have grown to love this client, but I can't be taken advantage of and/or manipulated like this.
>
> Please someone help me on how to deal with this situation. Please guide me on what steps I need to take, if any.

This was my response:

> Lauren; First, my sympathies. You sound fairly "beat up" by this situation. I have a few thoughts.
>
> The taking-care-of-yourself part: This is a perfect situation to learn from your own feelings and reactions (countertransference). If you are feeling resentful (and it sure sounds like it), this always means there is a request that you could have made or a "no" you

could have said before getting to this point. Are you truly OK with your late-cancellation policy? If your policy fits for you, you would not feel resentful when someone cancels. You might consider redesigning it (making it 48 or 72 hours, or charging more, or have a policy that is different for evening appointments) so when a client does not show, you are not thrown off and resentful.

You could also try the approach of relishing the paid time off when she cancels. Use it for professional or fun reading, cleaning up your desk or making phone calls.

<u>The part that belongs to the client:</u> She indeed may have issues about commitment to this work. Does she have a therapist? I would not recommend continuing to work with such a client unless she is seeing a therapist and you have a good working relationship with him or her. That would, I presume, be your approach with a client with a classic eating disorder. If she does have a therapist, I would talk with him or her about this issue of frequent cancellations. A therapist would call this a "clinical issue." In other words, it's not only annoying, but it's also meaningful and can be worked with. It's not your job alone to help the client work through her ambivalence. but you are in a wonderful position to work in tandem with the therapist to help the client see and accept her deeply mixed feelings. As a matter of fact, for many such clients, doing this work is central and essential if they are to address their overeating. (Here I am assuming she is a compulsive overeater.)

Finally, it is indeed difficult to keep separate your stuff and the client's stuff. Things go much smoother when you can. Do you have a supervisor to help you sort this out?

Language for Contact With Clients Who Don't Return

Most of these would work in either letter or phone format:

State what is true:
- You missed last week's appointment.
- I haven't heard from you about rescheduling that appointment you canceled.
- You are still below an adequate weight to support a healthy life.
- Your blood sugar is still in the range that leads to the complications of diabetes.
- It's hard to recover from an eating disorder and so it's tempting to run away from the process.
- I remember you told me that you left a dietitian in the past because ...
- I know this is a busy time of year for you.

State what you believe is the appropriate treatment:
- My experience is that it usually takes sessions twice a month for at least three months to adjust your food plan into one that works for you and keeps your blood sugar down.
- The most effective way to recover from an eating disorder is to work with a team.
- I don't believe it is wise to end treatment when your eating-disorder behaviors are still occurring.

Stay curious and leave the door open to future work:
- I'm not clear what has kept you from rescheduling and I'd be glad to talk about it.
- I would be glad to continue to work with you at any time.

Offer what you can do if the client returns:
- In future sessions. we could work more on ...
- I know we didn't get to discuss how to handle eating out. We could address that some other time if you'd like.
- We could attend more to specifically what you need.

Respect the client's choice:
- It's your choice whether to work with me.
- I hear that you have chosen to stop working on these goals.

* If you would prefer working with another nutritionist, I'd be glad to give you some referrals.

If appropriate, inform the client what action you are taking:
* I will send a letter to your doctor and your therapist letting them know you have ended with me.
* I will contact your doctor to let her know the limited progress we made with diet changes.

Self-Statements to Care for Yourself

* Of course I'm angry for the lost time/money. Now, how can I recoup a bit by using this time well?
* I've done my best with the client.
* Yes, I'm concerned for her health. Is there something appropriate for me to do here?
* I can't control what others choose to do or not do. I don't have to like that, but it's true.
* Since this is a professional relationship, the client doesn't owe me an explanation as a friend would.
* I prefer stories with endings and I get that from novels and movies. I can't expect to get it from my clients all the time.

Practice Steps: Handling Clients Who Don't Return

1. The next time a client seems to drop out of treatment, use the questions in the Tip to determine if follow-up is warranted.
2. If you decide to follow up, clarify what you want to say, using the suggestions above. Even if you do it by phone, it's handy to have an outline of your points written down.
3. If you decide not to follow up or get no response, move on to the self-care stage. Find a few statements above that feel supportive. Say them over a few times to link them to this case in your memory.

My Experiments With Handling Clients Who Don't Return

What I observe:

_____
_____
_____
_____
_____
_____
_____
_____
_____
_____
_____
_____
_____
_____
_____

How I will experiment:

_____
_____
_____
_____
_____
_____
_____
_____
_____
_____
_____
_____
_____
_____
_____
_____

Tip #25
Our Roles as Nutrition Therapists

Personally I'm always ready to learn,
although I do not always like being taught.
Sir Winston Churchill

The only ones among you who will be
really happy are those who will
have sought and found how to serve.
Albert Schweitzer

This is one of the Tips in which we **take a step back** and examine the process between us and our client. Is the role we take with a client working? Let's begin with the various roles we find ourselves in (or a client seems to wish us in). Here are some examples:

- Teacher of facts/provider of information/food guru
- Food police
- Sounding board/brainstorming and problem-solving partner
- Therapist for relationship with food/body
- Confessor/someone to be accountable to
- Cheerleader/motivator/coach
- Judge/moral adviser who tells client what is right and wrong
- Parent/nurturer
- Reality check
- Magician
- Debater
- Friend
- Role model

Criteria for choosing the role that fits for each client at each stage of work:

♦ **Fit your client's style:** An example is the familiar teacher role. Some clients thrive on the information you provide and can't get enough. Others can take only a little at a time and need you to ask them if they are ready for you to slip into that role for a while. Some clients look to you as a cheerleader and respond well when you praise their progress. Adjusting your role to what the client seems to want can be tricky. For example, a client may wish you to act as the food police because it is familiar and therefore comfortable. However, it may be just the setup that increases resistance to change. A comfortable role is not necessarily effective. Over the years, I have learned to refuse the food police role because it always backfires eventually.

♦ **Promote a professional relationship:** Some roles reinforce an appropriate professional relationship and some undermine it. We all want our clients to like us, and some would even make good friends. However, behaving with a client the way we do with a friend is inappropriate and lessens our effectiveness. (See Tips #1, Self-Disclosure; #13, Dual Relationships; and #18, Personal Questions, for more on professional boundaries.)

♦ **Effectiveness:** For clients who are resistant to change (the vast majority), review Tip #9, Dealing With Resistance. Resistance is less when we promote the client's choice and control, when we closely track readiness, and when we find ways to stop pushing and come alongside to work collaboratively. Which roles work *with* resistance and which make it worse? For example, allowing a client to use us as a judge (as some seem to want) works against the client's ability to make free choices and will to increase resistance.

♦ **Fitting in with other health professionals' roles:** Your role will vary depending on your work setting and the other team members' training and skills. For example, if you work with eating disorders, get to know the therapists with whom you share clients. One may welcome your work on the client's relationship with food if she carefully avoids all talk of food in therapy sessions. Another will prefer that you stay with nutrition education and provide only a reality check to the client's body and food beliefs.

Use your awareness of shifting roles to **direct the session**. When you feel uncomfortable with the role you find yourself in, learn from it. For example, your discomfort may alert you to the client's ambivalence to change. When I find myself arguing with a client, I know it's time to back off and revisit with the client her goals and what is most important to her. In other cases, your discomfort could allow you an opening to bring up the client's need for a therapist. For example, "Today it feels like I'm being your therapist. Since I'm not a trained psychotherapist, let's find you one. It sounds as if you are ready for therapy."

Learn to **shift roles flexibly.** In one session, you may need to move through several roles. You might first provide a reality check for distorted beliefs, then move to provide empathy for how hard change is, then educate about specific foods, then problem-solve with the client about how to make progress this week. If you find yourself almost entirely in one or two roles for most sessions, try on new ones as an experiment. For example, if you spend much of your time in the educator role, play with being a sounding board/problem-solving partner with all of your clients for the next week. Or if you tend to do lots of cheerleading, see what happens if you let that go for a while and simply provide empathy instead.

Be willing to **talk about roles in a treatment team.** If you feel confused or frustrated, your effectiveness is likely compromised. This is especially true in eating-disorder work in which clients may attempt to manipulate team members. Bring up with other team members your concerns about the role you find yourself in. In medical settings, your counseling for health behavior change is dependent on the support of others on the team. Make sure other professionals know what you can do and that they accurately convey this to clients.

Use supervision to examine which roles you and your client are in now and what might work better. Supervision is also a good setting to explore which roles you like best and slip into easily. You could ask for help expanding your capacity into a broader range of roles.

In summary, a useful guideline is to choose the role that allows you to stay both **client-centered and gently directive** at the same time.

Case Study: Losing Yourself With a Client

At a Counseling Intensive workshop, an experienced dietitian asked me about getting overly involved with clients. We had very little time left, and I felt the topic was too important to give a short answer. I asked her to call me a few weeks later, and we recorded the call. She wishes to remain anonymous, so her name has been changed.

Barbara: My question is about boundaries and getting overly empathetic with clients.

Molly: Would it help to look at a particular client?

Barbara: It might, but I should preface this by saying that this is something that I have been working on over many years in my own therapy.

Molly: In relationships with family members or with clients?

Barbara: Both. So my tendency is with anybody, client or not, it's all about them and there's nothing left there for me. Their needs are always more important than my needs.

Molly: And of course, Barbara, if that theme has come up for you in almost all your relationships, of course it would come up with clients, too. I'd be glad to see whether we can come up with ways to help you with clients. So far, over the years, what have you learned that has been useful?

Barbara: Well, I've learned that I have to stop and remember that I'm just as important as the next guy. The more I practice that, the better I've gotten at it.

Molly: Good. So when you remind yourself of this, you're able to hang on to yourself better and lose yourself less.

Barbara: Correct.

Molly: Do you have any really concrete ways to remember to do that, or phrases you say to yourself? I want to get an even clearer sense of what it is that works for you. Do you actually talk to yourself in your head or isn't it quite that? Is it more a thought or idea?

Barbara: It's not quite actually talking to myself in my head. It's just this intuition, this little red flag. Then I may actively say to myself, "All right, Barbara, be careful, remember not to lose

183

yourself here. Don't go in there so far. You have to make a boundary here. It's not your job to fix anything at this point. All you can do is facilitate."

Molly: You really have these phrases that work for yourself. Wow.

Barbara: I've been in therapy. It's like I have a supervisor and a therapist all rolled into one. I find that it starts to become all about somebody else or the feelings get so huge and I don't know what to do with them. I immediately take them to her, and we sort it out together.

Molly: So you use that relationship to help ground you.

Barbara: Absolutely, and for any dietitian who has never had the experience of being in therapy themselves, I would say, "Get thee to supervision! You will learn so much about yourself and then in turn be a better helper for your clients." I've learned that I can't help anybody if I get lost in their mess.

There are two clients that I have right now that still continue to push my buttons. They tend to be withholding and that pisses me off and I get into pushing them. I have figured out that they remind me of my mother.

Molly: The client puts you in a situation that is like the one you experienced with your mother and then you (of course) take on the role you did all those years ago and apply it in the session. This is likely not the role that will be most useful to the client. So, in therapy, you remind yourself that your mother and the client are two different people. Does this allow you to let go of the role you used to get into with your mother?

Barbara: Absolutely. I'm always very interested in hearing if other people experience this in their practice. Does this happen for you, Molly, and what do you do? Maybe you don't want to self-disclose about that.

Molly: I would be willing to briefly share because I hear you say this would be helpful. I can't say that I've had precisely the same experience. We're all different. The way I find myself losing myself tends to be by over-identifying with the client. For instance, if there's a college-age client and she's going through some things that remind me of what I went through at that age, it will grab me. I then may take on a specific role (advice-giving, for example) that I wanted at that age, but may not be right for this client.

Barbara: Right. That's part of what I mean by losing myself.

Molly: Let me ask you one other piece about this. My guess is, Barbara, that when you are talking about *process* with a client, it would be hard for you to lose yourself. In these moments, you're talking from what *you* know about working with other clients and what is in the literature. That's *you* speaking from what you know.

Barbara: Yes, and I do talk about my counseling philosophy with clients at times. I believe it's a team effort between the two people and the only reason I'm there is to guide the team. There may be a time when the client will guide us for a little while and I'm going along for the ride. What I used to do was just go off on the ride, but now I realize how important it is to keep me in the process, because if I don't, we may go off on this unstructured ride together.

Molly: Also, with eating-disordered clients, the eating disorder may be taking everybody for a ride, which, of course, doesn't do anybody any good. I hear that you've gotten better at hanging on to what you know to be true and to monitor the process based on your job, which includes attending to nutritional adequacy and medical health.

Barbara: Exactly.

Molly: So we've hit on another way to stay grounded. You can remind yourself that you're the dietitian in the room. You're the one who went to grad school, and is paid to hold the information and the perspective about health and nutrition that get lost in the client's eating disorder or anxiety or mood management. It can be your job to say, "Hello, we're forgetting something here."

Well, Barbara, I hope that you've gotten something out of this.

Barbara: Absolutely! Because hearing myself talk about it with you, I realize I am getting better at this. It's something I think I will always have to be aware of.

Practice Steps: Our Roles

1. Take a look at the list of roles in the Tip. Can you add some that you notice yourself taking?

2. Think back over the last few clients you saw and list all the roles you played. Do this for various types of clients.

3. Note any patterns. Do you tend to stay with one role for most of each session? Do some clients seem to encourage you to take a certain role? Which roles do you feel most comfortable with? Which are most uncomfortable?

4. Evaluate your habitual roles for effectiveness and appropriateness. You may find it helpful to talk this over with a colleague or supervisor.

5. If you find yourself using only a few roles, experiment with others less familiar to you. For example, to expand into the role of a sounding board, pick a client to do this with and shift into the process of just mirroring for a few minutes here and there in the session. See what happens. (For more on this process, review Tip #6, Mirroring.)

6. Realize you take on an inappropriate role at times? The supervision session in this section may guide you to move away from this role. If not, consult a supervisor.

7. Is there a role you find uncomfortable? This may be because it is indeed inappropriate for nutrition counseling or for this client. Or it may be uncomfortable because you are simply unaccustomed to it. You may need to talk this over with others to figure it out.

My Experiments With Roles

What I observe:

_____

_____

_____

_____

_____

_____

_____

_____

_____

_____

_____

_____

_____

_____

_____

_____

How I will experiment:

_____

_____

_____

_____

_____

_____

_____

_____

_____

_____

_____

_____

_____

_____

_____

_____

Suggested Reading List

Body Image:

"Body Wars: Making Peace With Women's Bodies" by Margo Maine

"Making Peace With Food: Freeing Yourself From the Diet/Weight Obsession" by Susan Kano

"Transforming Body Image: Learning to Love the Body You Have" by Marcia Hutchinson

Childhood Feeding:

"Child of Mine: Feeding With Love and Good Sense" by Ellyn Satter

"Secrets of Feeding a Healthy Family" by Ellyn Satter

"Your Child's Weight: Helping Without Harming" by Ellyn Satter

Eating Disorders:

"Anorexia Nervosa: A Guide to Recovery" by Lindsey Hall and Monika Ostroff

"Bulimia: A Guide to Recovery" by Lindsey Hall and Leigh Cohn

"Eating Problems: A Feminist Psychoanalytic Treatment Model" by Carol Bloom, Andrea Gitter, Susan Gutwill, Laura Kogel and Lela Zaphiropoulos

"Eating in the Light of the Moon" by Anita Johnston

"Eating Disorders: Nutrition Therapy in the Recovery Process" by Dan W. Reiff and Kathleen Reiff

"Surviving an Eating Disorder" by Michele Siegel and Judith Brisman

"The Eating Disorders Clinical Pocket Guide: Quick Reference for Healthcare Professionals" by Jessica Setnick, MS, RD

Health At Every Size Approach:

"Intuitive Eating" by Evelyn Tribole and Elyse Resch

"Moving Away From Diets: New Ways to Heal Eating Problems and Exercise Resistance" by Karin Kratina, Nancy L. King and Dayle Hayes

Health Behavior Change:

"Health Behavior Change" by Stephen Rollnick, Pip Mason and Chris Butler

"Moving Away From Diets: New Ways to Heal Eating Problems and Exercise Resistance" by Karin Kratina, Nancy L. King and Dayle Hayes

"Motivational Practice" by Rick Botelho

"Weighty Issues: Fatness and Thinness as Social Problems" edited by Jeffery Sobal and Donna Maurer

Sports Nutrition:

"Endurance Sports Nutrition" by Suzanne Girard Eberle

"Nancy Clark's Sports Nutrition Guidebook" by Nancy Clark

INDEX

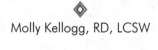

Contact Information

Molly Kellogg, RD, LCSW
100 East Sedgwick St.
Philadelphia, Pa. 19119
215-843-8258
www.mollykellogg.com
molly@mollykellogg.com

Services and Programs

Free Monthly E-mail Tips Series

The Counseling Tips continue!   Receive the new ones as I write them.
Subscribe on the Web site.

Counseling Intensive Training Workshop

This is a practical, nine-hour workshop offered around the country.   Using
a mix of presentation, practice with partners, video vignettes of client
sessions, and group discussion, this workshop will give you the confidence
you need. Check the Web site for the latest schedule.

> "This was the most motivating conference I have attended in
> years!!" **Jenny Favret, RD**

> "This was the missing piece! I'm excited to go back and
> start practicing! I'm so happy that you share your passion
> with other RD's!" **Mindy Ellsworth, RD**

> "Your seminar was one of the most valuable educational
> experiences of my career. I feel a completely different
> connection with my clients, and they are responding with
> great openness." **Judi LiVigni, MS, RD, CDN**

On-Site Staff Training

Invite me to design a program especially for your out-patient health team.

> "The workshop was great! It was exactly what our team needed and everyone clearly valued the experience. Your presentation skills are superb." **Helen M. Seagle, MS RD, Weight Management Program Director, Kaiser Permanente, Denver, CO**

> "This should be a required learning experience for the majority of nutrition professionals. Well, organized, well presented and interesting. This was the most enjoyable CE program I've been to in 10 years!" **Rick Weissinger, MS, RD, State of Delaware, Division of Public Health, School-Based Health Center Dietitian**

Phone Supervision

Sign up for group or individual supervision to get the tailored support you need. Details on the supervision page at www.mollykellogg.com.

> "You are wonderful to work with and have so much depth to your teachings." **Hien Nguyen-Le, RD**

> "What a gift you are to those of us in this field." **Jennie Wade, RD**

CPE Credits

I am a continuing professional education accredited provider with the Commission on Dietetic Registration. Credits for Registered Dietitians and Dietitian Technicians, Registered are approved for all trainings and group and individual supervision.